Journey into Power

How to Sculpt Your Ideal Body,

Free Your True Self,

and Transform Your Life

with Yoga

Journey

into Power

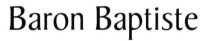

Baron Baptiste

Photographs by Richard Corman

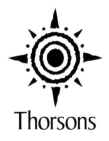

Thorsons

Thorsons
An Imprint of HarperCollins*Publishers*
77-85 Fulham Palace Road,
Hammersmith, London W6 8JB

The Thorsons website address is: www.thorsons.com

and *Thorsons*

are trademarks of HarperCollins*Publishers* Ltd

First published in the US by Fireside, an Imprint of Simon & Schuster 2002
This edition published by Thorsons 2002

10 9 8 7 6 5 4 3 2 1

Photographs by Richard Corman

A catalogue record of this book is available from the British Library

ISBN 0 00 713328 6

Printed and bound in Italy by Editoriale Johnson SpA

This publication contains the opinions and ideas of its author. It is intended to provide helpful and informative material on the subjects addressed in the publication. It is sold with the understanding that the author and publisher are not engaged in rendering medical, health, or any other kind of professional services in the book. The reader should consult his or her medical, health, or other competent professional before adopting any of the suggestions in this book or drawing inferences from it.

The author and publisher specifically disclaim all responsibility for any liability, loss or risk, personal or otherwise, which is incurred as a consequence, directly or indirectly, of the use and application of any of the contents of this book.

Acknowledgments

This book was a journey traveled by an incredible team made up of people who never accepted that something was impossible.

I am deeply grateful for their efforts through many late days and long hours. We have all grown and become more in the process.

Thanks to my parents for everything you've given me, and to my two sisters, Sherri and Devi, for always standing by me. Thanks to D'ana Baptiste for instilling love and meaningful values into the boys. I thank God for giving me the ability to spend generous amounts of time with my children. My favorite place to be is with my three boys, who bring a depth and joy to my life that soars way beyond words.

A huge thank you to my literary agent, Ling Lucas, who has maintained a protective and loving eye over the creation of this book. I am deeply grateful for your vision, tenacity, and true belief in this work.

I thank Debra Goldstein, my gifted wordsmith who faithfully followed me around the world. To me, you are a great sculptor who skillfully and patiently helped me to shape the lifetime of information that is found within the pages of this book.

To my incredible editor, Caroline Sutton: Your vision, passion, commitment, and constant encouragement brought all of the components of this book together in a really wonderful way. Thank you for being so present.

A big thank you to Kate Churchill, who helped bring this book to completion. Your contribution was enormous, and your vision combined with follow-through makes it clear to me that the completion of this book is not the end of anything; it is just the beginning.

To Coeli Marsh for sharing her beautiful yoga practice in the pictures of this book. Thank you for your commitment, support, and hard physical work during a long and adventurous photo shoot that took place during a tropical hurricane.

A heartfelt thanks to Richard Corman and his trusted assistant Peter Chin, who faithfully ventured to meet me on a tropical island paradise and shoot the photos in this book. Your pictures are a testimony to your skill and unending composure.

Thank you to Mark Gompertz, Trish Todd, Chris Lloreda, Debbie Model, Cherlynne Li, Marcia Burch, Laurie Cotumaccio, Nicole Diamond, and the other members of the Fireside team who supported me and worked crazy hours behind the scenes day and night to bring this book into the world.

To my entire teaching team at the Baptiste Power Yoga Institute in Cambridge, Boston, and Philadelphia, who diligently carry forth this powerful work and maintain the integrity of the vision. The significance of your contribution is proven in the gratitude that shines back to you from the eyes of the thousands of people who come through our studios each week. I bow to you.

A hundred salutations to the hundreds of students who have graduated from my teacher training Bootcamps and are spreading this work around the world like wildfire, and especially to Bill Raup and Rhea Schlicter for your work in keeping Baptiste yoga ablaze in your bustling studios in the Philadelphia area.

Rolf and Mariam Gates, I bow to you guys and your burning enthusiasm that keeps the Baptiste Power Yoga Institute in Boston and Cambridge spirited and thriving.

To Mark Aronchik for your unending guidance, support, and friendship, I thank you.

Thank you to the Kennedy clan, who have supported this work, and specifically to Max and Vicki Kennedy, who were influential in moving my family from Philadelphia to Boston. I will always cherish the days spent at Hyannis Port with our families and sailing together in Cape Cod.

To Jeffrey and Christina Lurie for bringing my family and me from Beverly Hills to Philadelphia. The years I spent as a part of the Philadelphia Eagles coaching staff were a monumental life experience for me that I will always hold as valuable. To you, I am eternally grateful.

A huge thank you to some of the most outstanding NFL coaches and athletes in the world: Ray Rhodes, John Gruden, Bill Romanowski, Randall Cunningham, Irving Fryar, Hershel Walker, Mike Mamula, Gary Anderson, Tommy Hutton, Rodney Peete, Jay Fiedler, The Refrigerator Perry, Charlie Garner, and Ricky Watters. The years I spent working with you guys taught me about character, discipline, and determination. Also, my Peak Performance Program with the Philadelphia Eagles was a success because of the enormous support and effort of my trusted assistant Bill Mancini.

Thanks to Helen Hunt, Elisabeth Shue, Chynna Phillips, Lolita Davidovich,

Holly Robinson Peete, and Raquel Welch, all of whom have supported this work now and/or in the past. Your contributions have impacted the quality of people's lives.

Thank you to my friend and spiritual brother Jesse Peterson whose constant love, rugged honesty, and inner knowledge have taught me a lot about the true meaning of the word *friend*. The constant commitment and selfless contribution you and your nonprofit organization B.O.N.D. are producing is truly making a difference.

Thank you to my best friend, David Masters, and your father, Roy. You guys are giants whose shoulders I stand upon. I salute you.

I am so grateful to my loyal and steadfast managers at BPYI offices and studios, who faithfully work day in and day out to bring me into workshops, Bootcamps, and classrooms across the continent that are overflowing with enthusiastic students. Hugh Folkerth and Jeanne Coffey are two dynamic dynamos who always stay committed to the vision that what we are doing does make a difference and that by helping our students grow to new levels, we grow as people.

I acknowledge and bow to the teachers who have guided me to my own understanding.

And most of all thanks to every person who has ever attended my classes, workshops, Bootcamps, or purchased a video or CD. Those who have shared with me the powerful testimony of the value that this work has had in their lives give us all the reasons to continue on our journey. Your support for this work means more to me than I could possibly put into words.

I dedicate this book to my two fathers, who are in heaven,
and to my three beautiful boys, Luke, Jacob, and Malachi. You are the giants in my life.

Contents

Journey
into Power

"Sculpt your ideal body . . . free your true self . . . transform your life . . ."

If I seem to be making a lot of promises to you here, that's because I am. It may sound too good to be true, but if you work the principles in this book, I guarantee you will journey into power in every area of your life. Your body will transform, you will change your destructive patterns permanently at a cellular level, your mind will be infused with life and equanimity, and your relationships will be truer, deeper, and more fulfilling.

How do I know this? Because I have seen thousands of students come through my studios, Bootcamps, and workshops and with my own eyes witnessed their transformations. I have seen students arrive the first night of Bootcamps anxious and heavy with emotional baggage, but by the time they leave, it's as if they have shed a hundred pounds of physical and psychic debris. I have witnessed overweight people who come to my studios create entirely new bodies within only a few months.

Countless students from all over the world who come to my programs write to me and tell me about breakthroughs they have experienced in all different areas of their lives—even those who have been practicing yoga for years! A forty-seven-year-old woman from Seattle wrote to tell me how she experienced a physical opening in her shoulders that created a tremendous release of old stress and sorrow that she had been carrying around with her for decades. She told me she hadn't felt this free since she was in her twenties! Another student, a thirty-six-year-old woman who teaches yoga in Colorado and has been doing yoga for nearly six years, e-mailed to say that she saw for the first time how her competitive nature was interfering with her growth and her overall happiness. She wrote: "I was able to see that I can challenge myself to my new heights . . . that yoga isn't about competition or comparison, but rather it is about pushing myself beyond my current abilities and moving past the limited definitions of myself."

People with lifelong aches tell me their pains have vanished after only a few practice sessions. Hundreds with chronic back problems experience quick and long-lasting relief and are able to resume activities they hadn't been able to do for many years. A twenty-two-year-old man who was going through a depression and did not want to take pills came to a workshop on the advice of his therapist. He stayed with his power yoga practice after that workshop, and within three months, the depression was totally gone. I have one student whose ovarian cancer went into remission after she wholly dedicated herself to a healing yoga practice.

Many others are inspired to make bold and wonderful changes in their lives, from leaving unhealthy relationships to venturing into careers they had always dreamed about. A very successful thirty-three-year-old systems analyst came to a Bootcamp looking for a change in her life, and on the last day she announced to all of us that she was going home with a newfound confidence and courage to quit the job she hated and go back to school to pursue her dream. She had simply opened herself up to whatever spontaneous insights would arise, and when this plan materialized, she knew in an instant that her life was about to take an amazing, wonderful turn.

But the main reason I am so convinced that my power yoga can transform people is that it happened to me. I didn't just arrive as a master yoga teacher, happy and serene, walking my authentic path. Like so many other people, I had to go through the dark to get to the light.

My parents, Walt and Magana Baptiste, were two of America's yoga pioneers. My father came from a fitness background (he was Mr. America in 1949), and in 1952 he and my mother were the first to open a yoga and health center in San Francisco. They were way ahead of their time as early proponents of the whole healthy lifestyle movement. From the time I was a little boy, yoga was part of my life. We had famous spiritual masters coming through our home all the time, from the Maharishi to Yogananda. It all seemed normal to me. While other kids were playing baseball and hanging out on the weekends, I would be off at my parents' spiritual and health retreat ranch in Sonoma Valley, watching people going through personal transformations and self-renewal programs. Back then, I just thought yoga was kind of fun, but not really a big deal. And *definitely* not how I would spend my life.

I hit my rebellious stage at around twelve years old. I started wanting to be with my friends on the weekends, not riding goats and meditating out on the farm. I got teased a lot at school, as you can imagine. The other kids would call me "Hare Krishna" and laugh when I brought banana and honey sandwiches on whole-wheat bread for lunch instead of lunch-meat and Twinkies. As you can imagine, my childhood was difficult, because at that point in American culture, I didn't fit in.

My rebelliousness was not just a result of not fitting in. I had a curious mind and a searching spirit that simply did not respond to being stuffed with school lessons and information that had no meaning to me. I was always questioning my teachers, because I knew there was something more out there than what the teachers were telling me. I had a huge appetite for growth and discovery, so I moved on to become a student of life.

I managed my father's health food restaurant to make enough money to travel around the world and surf. I went to Mexico, Bali, Asia, and, when I needed a rest, to my parents' retreat center in Central America, which was filled with amazing and interesting people who shared my quest for knowledge and a deeper understanding of life. I was drawn there more and more, and it eventually became a kind of home base for me, a place where I could come into contact with other soul searchers.

Around that time I started reading stories about the prophets and sages, about Jesus, Buddha, Socrates, and Gandhi. I read Yogananda's famous book, *Autobiography of a Yogi,* and was fascinated by his vivid, magical descriptions of being in the light and the philosophies of the mystics of old. It made me yearn to find my own path to bliss—my own inner light.

So I began a spiritual search that lasted for many years. I made a choice to go for it, and to really seek out the enlightenment I had been reading about, I moved to Yogananda's men's ashram in Encinitas, California. We did kriya yoga (based on chakra energy), meditated, and worked on the farm, all in silence. I stayed at the ashram for about a year, and though it was a very introspective time, I still felt empty. I just wasn't finding the bliss all the books were talking about. The more I learned about the yoga tradition, the less it seemed to speak to me. It was all more confusing than ever, and true life mastery started to seem unattainable. I got very proficient at my practice and experienced some benefits, but somehow it just wasn't all coming together.

After I left the ashram, I went back up to my parents' studio and worked part-time in their health food store. One afternoon my father asked me to fill in for him at a yoga and meditation class he had scheduled. I didn't want to do it, but he pressed me and told me I knew a lot and I had a lot to share from my experiences. He told me I had a responsibility to share what I knew, that if you don't share it you lose it. Sharing what you know makes it more real, more a living part of you. I reluctantly agreed, and to my surprise, teaching came very naturally to me. I just opened my mouth and spoke about what I knew, and the students loved it. I couldn't believe it. That was the first time it had ever dawned on me that perhaps I would make teaching yoga my life.

Around my nineteenth birthday, the hatha yoga master B. K. S. Iyengar came to San Francisco from India, and it was at his workshop that I first witnessed the powerfully physical side of yoga that went beyond any of the forms I had practiced up until then. I had always been athletic (I had been studying martial arts since I was nine years old; by the time I was eighteen I had earned my black belt and won the California State Championship title for tae kwon do), so what Iyengar was teaching was exciting to me in a whole new way.

A couple of years later, when Bikram Choudhury (founder of Bikram yoga) came and taught a workshop in San Francisco, he invited me to move to Los Angeles and be his protégé. I was curious about Los Angeles, and it seemed time to leave San Francisco, so I went and studied with Bikram, and within about a year I was teaching his style of yoga, also intensely physical. My body became incredibly strong and flexible as I became very good at contorting it into demanding poses, but my spirit was still restless. I had tried the ashram route, but that didn't give me the answers. Now I was being taught that if I could just get all the poses right, I would be enlightened. I was getting them right, but though I did feel a certain level of vitality, something was still missing.

I continued on this way for a few years, teaching at Bikram's studios in Beverly Hills and Paris, and studying with Iyengar and others in India. By all outward appearances I was "yoga-ing" right: I followed the advice of the gurus, practiced daily, was a vegetarian, didn't drink any alcohol or do any drugs. But my relationships weren't working, and inside I felt at a loss and, most of all, empty. There was still a big block within. Being able to meditate for six straight hours or wrap my legs around my head or hold a handstand longer didn't necessarily change me on a deeper level. Like so many other people, I hit the bottom of my soul and really wondered: Is this all there is?

Looking back now I see that I was in a waking sleep, a mild hypnosis. Even though I was practicing yoga and meditation, I was misusing it; cultural conditioning had taught me to stay distracted and anesthetized and not to see or feel what was really happening within me, both the good and the bad. Somehow all the mind/body "medicine" I was learning was falling short of a cure.

The day it all started to turn around for me began like any other day. I was in Los Angeles, on my way home from teaching one of my now-popular classes at the famous Voight Fitness and Dance Center in Hollywood (where Johnny G. was launching spinning in the next room). I'd been teaching there for a few years, taking traditional yoga practices and making them empowering and accessible to all types of people. I was putting this all into a flow practice that was more athletic than the styles I'd been taught, and it was catching on in a huge way. I had become the "yoga teacher to the stars" and achieved a certain level of celebrity. From the outside it looked as if I had it all, but inside myself I knew there had to be more. All the success wasn't filling the void, and the mechanics of yoga just weren't cutting it for me anymore. There was a big piece missing, but I simply didn't know where to look.

Anyway, that afternoon, I heard a spiritual psychologist speaking on the radio. He was saying that the only way to find true peace, acceptance, and power was through stillness. He said that being in stillness leads you to truth, but you may not always like to see and hear the truth, because very often it isn't the rosy picture you might have hoped for. Something exploded within me when I heard that. Maybe I was finally open enough to see it, but the truth unfolded for me in that moment like never before. I realized that the truth I could not admit was that I was simply regurgitating what others were teaching me. I was filled with the advice and teachings of gurus and books, but had no idea what *I* really thought or felt. I'd spent my entire life up until that point looking outward, seeking inner peace like it was a goal, never really daring to come face-to-face with the truth that was within me.

This speaker broke through to me in a way that all those years of chanting and meditating and twisting my body into a pretzel never had, and that was because he was the first to truly ignite my spirit. It was in that moment that I realized how severely I had neglected my authentic self—my inner voice—my real wisdom. I went home that day and cried, because I saw myself deeply and clearly for the first time. I saw all of my unfinished business in the forms of resentment, fear, withholding of forgiveness, anger, jealousy, insecurities, and self-doubt, and saw how I had been working to just stuff it down with "feel good" pseudospirituality. I had been looking toward mastery of the practices and paths of others instead of paying respect to and honoring what was already within me. I saw that if I stopped smothering my spirit and soul with external knowledge goals, I would actually start feeling, and ultimately healing.

Knowing and accepting these truths started to finally set me free. I saw where I was being dishonest with others, and started being more honest about how and who I was in every moment. I began to unravel all the emotional knots that had been strangling me. My revelation was that my true path was to more deeply accept that which I already knew and had within me. I realized there was a power that would give me peace—that yoga practice offers valuable tools but only insofar as they lead to one's inner self.

As a teacher, I started seeing that we don't have to take dogma so seriously. When we start to take it too seriously, outer mastery becomes the goal, and we are then chasing the illusion once again. Spiritual masters often teach that tradition is holy, and that we must follow it to the letter if we are to be enlightened. Do it their way or it won't work. But how can that be? If we tune out the inner voice of wisdom in favor of what someone else is telling us, how can we ever really be in our own power? That just puts us in the shadows of someone else's power, of someone else's courage to look within for the answers. It was only then that I was able to start teaching with real integrity and began to share with my students that we must each find and walk our own path.

This focus on intuition rather than tradition hit a nerve with many of my students and formed the core philosophy of what was later to become Baptiste Power Vinyasa Yoga. Attendance at my classes exploded, and new students began appearing every day. I was at last fully present in a way I had never been. They came because they wanted beautiful bodies, but they stayed because they were inspired to be the best versions of themselves. They had listened to all the others, walked the paths, but ultimately discovered the same thing I did: The only person who can open the door to the inner truths and lead you to the light is yourself.

Ultimately, no yoga teacher can tell you what you need—not in a pose, not in a diet, not in a lifestyle. They can give you the principles, but it is up to you to use your intuition to find what is right for you. You have to practice your own naturalness, and that is what Baptiste Power Yoga is all about.

I will share with you the ancient pillars of life that will illuminate your journey. I will show you how to access the innate wisdom in your mind, the strength and suppleness in your body, the infinite and exquisite beauty of your spirit. But ultimately, I'm not teaching you anything you don't already know somewhere deep within your being. Your genetic systems are encoded with this knowledge. My role is to awaken you to what you have simply forgotten along the way.

I feel honored and blessed to be your guide on your own personal Journey into Power, and I hope this program brings you all the joy and fulfillment it has brought me.

Namaste,
Baron Baptiste
Cambridge, Massachusetts
September 2001

Introduction

Welcome to power yoga—the ultimate wake-up call!

So many of us are striving so hard to be better, to know more, do more, be more. We have been conditioned to believe that we are not good enough the way we are. We're afraid that if we do less, we'll be less, so we read all the latest self-improvement books, take the seminars, follow the diets, go to the gym, but nothing seems to really get us where we want to go. We still weigh too much, worry too much, and race around searching for something that will soothe whatever it is that we see as our problem.

But I believe we all have just one problem. Yes, you read that right: Every single one of us is suffering from the same problem. Of course, your life looks different from mine, or your friend's, or your neighbor's. You might even think your problems are completely unique, but for those of us who feel dissatisfied with our bodies or our lives, there is only one expla-

nation: We are not living from our authentic selves, from our truth. We are asleep to who and what we really are and can be.

We blame external factors for our woes—our parents, our careers, our hectic lives, our spouses, our thighs, our lack of time to exercise or eat right—but the only thing that is "wrong" with us or our lives is that we are disconnected from our core. We were programmed to believe that things like status, money, achievement, and a perfect body would make us happy, or better yet, a complete person. We were taught that these goals were more important than honoring our authentic nature; the timeless and universal truths within us. The question is, are material possessions and perfect abs and thighs the object of our real search? We're pursuing some better version of ourselves, all the while asleep to the one true fact in the universe: Our ideal selves are already within us, just waiting to be awakened. Our only task is to relinquish the luggage of life and accept what was there from the start: the light in our hearts and the power within.

Michelangelo used to say that God put a statue within every slab of marble, and his job was to remove all that was not part of the statue. He claimed he merely freed the statue from the stone. I have studied and practiced yoga for nearly my entire life, and I know that it can be a powerful tool to help you free your own personal "statue." That is why I teach and why I have written this book. Because beneath the habits of our materialistic lifestyles and the stresses and demands of maintaining the identity we have created lie our true selves and the deeper meaning of life. I want to share with you how to peel away the layers that keep your magnificent body and inner being from shining through.

Journey into Power is not about seeking the answers from some outside source. It's not about piling on muscles, or gaining more knowledge, or finding a better relationship. You have been taught your whole life to look outside yourself, to parents, teachers, experts, maybe even to gurus, but all you need is already within you. It's time we wrap our arms around that truth! The goal here is not to go out and find yourself, for you were never really lost. Forgotten maybe, but not lost.

Journey into Power is about excavating the amazing, radiant self already inside you. Within you is a power that is already perfect, and the true essence of *seeking* on this journey is *accepting.* Your greatest power, your greatest wisdom, your greatest en-

lightenment is not suddenly going to appear in ten or twenty years. It's already here. Like Michelangelo's statues, within each of us lies our authentic body and our natural, divine self; all we need to do is chisel away all that does not belong in order to reveal it. And that is where my yoga program comes in.

Yoga is ultimately a journey into truth: truth about who you really are, what you are capable of, how your actions affect your life. Truth is the only medicine that ever "cures" us; it is the only means by which we can live at our full, incredible potential. At the most basic level, so many of us are not living life at 100 percent. But if you are not living in truth, you are cheating yourself. If you are living in a body that is weighed down and unhealthy, you are robbing yourself of your vitality. If you are plagued by anxiety and worry, you are denying yourself the peace that is so readily available to you. If you are controlled by your fears and emotions, you have sacrificed your personal power.

We could all be playing at a much greater level if we would only dare to go beyond where we are stuck. That's what yoga tells and shows us. Down through the ages, every great teacher has taught that we have the ultimate power to break through and therefore "break with" that which holds us back.

On the first night of Bootcamps I tell the students that I'm going to squeeze them like oranges. If you squeeze an orange, you get orange juice, so my question to them is "If we squeeze you, what will we get?" That's what this process of yoga does. It wrings you from the inside out. It brings up everything that's in there—the fears, doubts, frustrations, toxins, strengths, beliefs, potential—and exposes it either to be released or to be used for growth. It challenges physically, emotionally, mentally, and spiritually and gives you the opportunity to experience every part of yourself on a whole new level.

It all starts in your body, on the mat. I'll show you how to turn back the clock and come alive like never before. One of my students, a professional athlete, recently called me to say how thrilled he was that his body had a strong tingling sensation all over.

"What's so thrilling about that?" I asked, curious to hear his take on it.

"My body hasn't been alive like that since I was eighteen years old!" he said. He was in touch with a body that had been lost to him since he was a boy. His body was an athletic machine, but he had become numb. Now he could feel again. The yoga practices in this book will allow you to do the same thing: to heal and to empower.

Power vinyasa yoga is an amazing form of fitness that sculpts strong, healthy bodies. The results are dramatic because it is a whole body system, using full body movements that encourage the body to move as nature intended. Because every single muscle is used in strength and balance, it ignites the metabolic furnace. It tones and chisels through isometrics and isotonics. You lose weight because active muscle tissue burns fat—the stronger your muscles are, the stronger your metabolic fire burns—and also because you won't have the same need to feed your fears and soothe your anxious edges by overeating. Within the first few practice sessions, your belly will get flatter, your buttocks tighter, your arms will get toned and strong, and you will tingle and sparkle from your temples to your toes. You will feel strong and calm, more energized and alive. You will begin to see your body taking on a shape and level of agility you have never experienced before. You will stand taller and look sleeker, straighter, and leaner. In time, you will awaken in a whole new body.

But the physical changes are only a byproduct of a more empowering purpose. The physical magic just kind of happens as you go through the practice. The real miracle is what starts happening underneath, within you.

We soak up life like a sponge, holding tensions, fears, and anxieties in our system. In yoga practice you reach down into all the nooks and crannies and hidden pockets of tissue, excavating all this clogging, unwanted stuff. Through the challenges on your mat, you step up to what I call your edge and pull up whatever is inside you that needs to be healed and released. You also discover how strong you really are, physically and mentally. Almost as if by magic, lifelong fears dissipate, blocked emotions are released, your mind gets quiet and gains startling clarity, psychic wounds from deep down surface to be healed. You experience mental shifts that free you from old thought patterns. You begin to understand on a deep level what is right for you and what to do. You just *get it.* These insights and revelations crystallize as something permanent and real within you.

At the same time, because it strips away all the excess debris, yoga brings you back to your sweetness, your innocence. It reminds you of your love of discovery. Children have natural yoga bodies because they haven't piled on the layers of toxic living, reactiveness, resentments, guilt, and anxiety that adults have. They have no blocks yet to stand in their way, and instinctively live from the center of their beings. My eight-year-old son has lots of friends, but when I once asked him who his very best friend was, he said, "Myself." As children we were complete within ourselves, but over the years we have come to live unnaturally. Yoga is a remarkably effective "unlearning" process. We have to unlearn our negative thought systems, our emotional patterns, our patterns of moving, breathing, and eating so that we can come back to our own naturalness.

On a deeper level, you awaken to cause and effect. You begin to have a meaningful understanding that every action you take generates a result. You see that what you put out there dictates what you get in return. If you are not putting out abundance, it's no wonder abundance is not pouring into your life! You start to connect the dots and recognize how the smallest daily actions have a domino effect. It hits you how

your overreactions to stress cause your negative eating habits, and how they in turn affect your body and energy levels. You start seeing clearly the things you are doing to limit or hurt yourself, and the ways you can grow. You see how launching into reactivity, anger, fear, or jealousy fuels vicious cycles in your relationships, and where your responsibility lies. You really start to *get it* that your life circumstances are the sum total of decisions you made along the way, and that the only person who can ultimately transform your life is you, by operating from the deeper level of cause rather than trying to struggle with the surface effects.

If you were to ask ten people, "What would you ask for if you were granted only one wish?" the answers would vary. One might say "a new car." Someone else might say "good health," "a happy relationship," or "a perfect body." Another may say "money." But these people would be blindly limiting their opportunities in life. If we were truly inclined toward fulfillment, peace of mind, and contentment, we would choose quite differently. We might say, "If I had one wish, I would wish that every good thing I ever wished for would come true." Here we would be using our one wish as the foundation for all other wishes.

We all have that choice in life. In yoga practice we learn that the first step toward everything worthwhile is consciously responding from our underlying foundation of truth in each moment. When you awaken to this, you begin to live more consciously and at cause in other areas of your life: your diet, your health, your relationships, your career, your money. Your bad habits and negative patterns will dissolve like snow in the summer sun.

Ultimately, yoga ignites your spirit. When you are free from the constraints of a weak body and the limitations of emotional reactiveness, you live in a higher place. You begin to dwell in spirit, and from there, all that remains that is not authentically you falls away. You carry an inner oasis of calm and composure, even in the midst of the chaos of daily living. The word *charisma* was originally a spiritual term meaning "gift of grace," and this is what you will radiate. People around you will notice the changes and say you are so lucky, but you will know that luck had nothing to do with it.

When you live from spirit, growth becomes the most important thing to you. Your desire to know and evolve—to take a fearless inventory of yourself—sharpens, and from there your path continues to unfold to infinity. Once you discover how empowering it is to live from your truth, there is no stopping you! It is no longer a question of "How can I grow?" but "How far do I want to go?"

The program in this book is based on my "Journey into Power" Bootcamps, which are intensive, seven-day programs designed to purify your body, rewire your mind, recharge your spiritual batteries, and awaken your inner power. Of course, I know not everyone has the time or re-sources to be able to leave their life behind for a week and dedicate themselves wholly to growth, so the purpose of this program is to take the practices from the Bootcamps and permanently incorporate them into a long-term life plan. This program can work for anyone at any age, any weight, any fitness level. I have seen it work for eighteen-year-olds and eighty-year-olds, all different body types, weights, and levels of strength and flexibility. From absolute beginners to people who have been practicing yoga for twenty years, this program truly works, if you work it.

The program has five parts:

Rewiring Your Mind
Daily Power Yoga Practice
The Cleansing Diet
Meditation for Truthful Living
Journeying into Real Life

The "Daily Power Yoga Practice" is the heart of the program. I encourage you to embrace the whole program for the most effective and fastest transformation, but even if you do nothing else but roll out your mat and do the yoga flow, you will see and feel the magic, miracles, and results. The other parts of the program are all master keys to transformation to which you will naturally gravitate once you begin to awaken. As old habits and patterns dissolve, they release you. Effortlessly and very naturally you will start thinking better, eating better, meditating (to cultivate stillness and insight), and taking your practice to the next level by living your yoga. If your spirit is ready for growth and you are really willing to part once and for all with what's not working for you, then take action and get on board for the whole program and total life transformation.

If you sense arrogance, know that it is not part of me or my teaching style. It comes from faith in the power of this process, which has worked for thousands of years and millions of students. Something does not stick around for five millennia if it doesn't work. I have simply taken the practice and simplified, demystified, and developed it into the ultimate accessible body and soul path for you to get the most out of life—right here, right now!

The first part, "Rewiring Your Mind," is where it all starts. Yoga teaches you to manage your mental and emotional states, and this shift originates in your mind. As you set forth on your new practice and begin peeling away the layers that you've worn as a defense for so many years, it helps to pay attention to the signals your mind is sending. We all have negative beliefs we buy into, most of which we don't even know about because they are so deeply ingrained in our subconscious. When you are spiritually asleep, these beliefs run your life. When you awaken, however, you open the window to new possibilities.

The timeless principles I introduce here are cues to assist you in your physical practice, but each also has a deeper meaning that you may find helpful in the context of your personal growth and everyday

life. Pick and choose what resonates for you at first, but revisit this section often to see if other principles take on new meaning for you as your practice deepens. I have worked these principles for many years and yet I still find fresh, new meaning in them with every new stage of growth.

Part Two, "Daily Power Yoga Practice," is where you will learn everything you need to know in order to start a power yoga practice at home. I will tell you what you need and what to expect. We'll talk about each posture in depth—how to do it, its transformational power, and more. You'll learn why it is important to practice daily, even if only for a few minutes; how to use the foundations of heat, breath, and flow; and how to create practices to fit into your schedule.

As a physical workout, power yoga is athletic yoga, so be prepared to sweat! It is unlike any other form of physical exercise you've ever done. It is challenging, but the beauty of it is that each person can adapt it to suit his or her own body. So even if you are just a beginner who has never even heard of the Sun Salutations, you will be able to do it. Each body will take the poses differently, and as you go through your practice you will begin to know when to push and when less is more, when to go for it and when to rest. When you are fully present in your physical practice, you will know what your body needs.

Part Three is "The Cleansing Diet." It's not a rigid regimen with weird recipes to follow. It's just the basic tenets of a health-giving, cleansing diet and the psychology behind it. Almost all of my students make changes in their eating once they begin doing power yoga. They start to feel lighter and cleaner, and lose the desire for their old unhealthy ways of eating. They now look for foods and habits that enhance their newfound vitality. You'll learn all about the hypnotic power of food and how to break its spell through mindful eating, why it's so important to eat water-rich foods, what "whole" foods are and why your body needs them, and how to let your negative eating habits fly away with the wind.

Part Four, "Meditation for Truthful Living," is where you will learn to cultivate stillness in your life. You've probably been told that meditation is good for you; what I will show is exactly why meditation is perhaps the single most important thing you can do for yourself every day. A regular meditation practice brings a powerful dimension to power yoga as it routinely empties your mental and emotional cup. It removes yesterday's stuff from your mind, cleaning the slate so you can continually return to your center and live in the now that is always fresh, new, and full of discovery.

A lot of people think meditation must mean sitting cross-legged and chanting "Om." Certainly that is one way to meditate, but I'll give you a painless and profoundly simple meditation technique from which you can benefit for the rest of your life. In fact, you'll wonder how you ever managed without it. The strength of coming into stillness will open new doors to you.

The last part of the book, "Journeying into Real Life," puts all you've learned into action. It includes ways to incorporate power yoga into your life and gives you tips on how to take your power yoga practice to the next level. You will learn how to make your practice a priority, things to remember when you find yourself going astray, and, ultimately, how to shine forth and make positive and healing changes in the world around you.

As I've said many times before, neither I nor any other teacher can tell you what is right for you. What I offer here are principles that have worked for many others, all of whom have in some way adapted the program so that it works for them. Don't follow me, follow yourself. I encourage you to dedicate yourself to your own growth, and use what resonates for you in this program to guide you along the way. Take what speaks to you and throw out what doesn't. Ultimately, it is *your* unique and personal path, not mine or anyone else's.

I promise that if you apply these timeless tools, your life will transform. The psychic debris will clear, your body will become strong and fit, and your spirit will be awakened. Your ultimate power is always within you; all you have to ask is "Am I willing to go for it?" and "If not now, when?" Your Journey into Power begins just by taking that most difficult first step, and you are already on your way just by picking up this book.

Welcome to the world of bliss. Now let's begin!

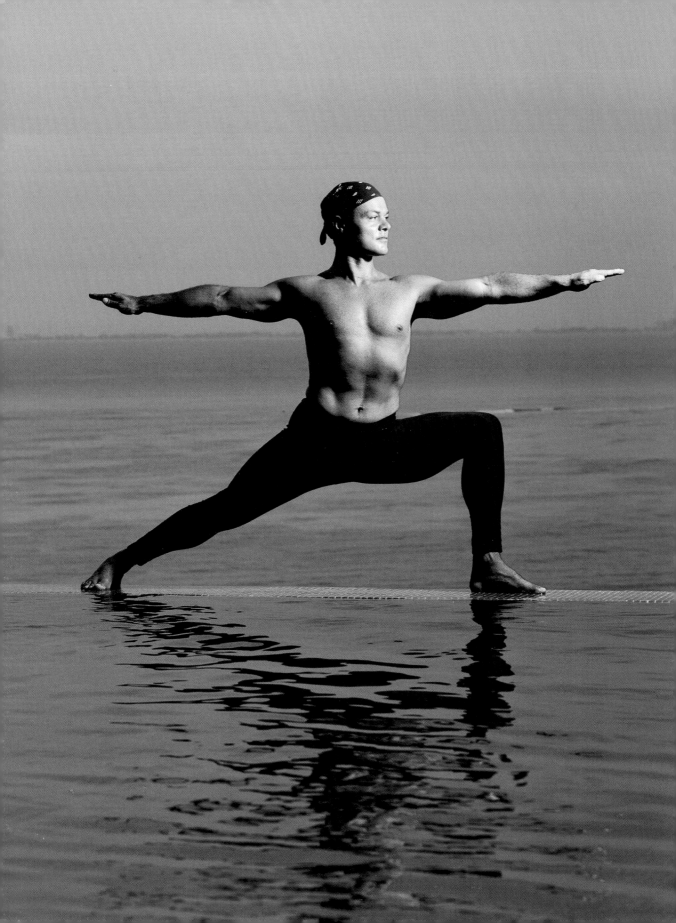

As we think and act, so our world becomes.

—The Dhammapadda

PART I

Rewiring

Your Mind

Where Transformation Begins

YEARS AGO, I WAS THE PRIVATE YOGA
TEACHER FOR A VERY WEALTHY MAN. HE WAS A BILLION-
AIRE WHO CAME FROM AN EXTREMELY POOR BACKGROUND WHO HAD

built his fortune from the ground up using nothing but intuition, common sense, and determination. One day I asked him how he had learned to create so much from so little, considering where he came from.

"Technique was only twenty percent of it," he told me. "The other eighty percent was my worldview."

Imagine that: Only 20 percent of success is the mechanics of achievement; the other 80 percent comes from your psychology. That idea has stayed with me ever since I heard it, because I can really see how true it is for everything in life. The "how to" element isn't the problem. It's how receptive we are to growth that really

determines how far we can go. It all comes down to whether we choose to play small or big, whether we become instruments of peace and power or vehicles for pain in this world.

The reason it is so difficult for us to change is that we focus too much on the microcosmic steps, or the "program," and not enough on changing the perspective that landed us where we are in the first place. Deep and true changes come from the inside out, not the other way around.

We can try all different kinds of techniques to transform ourselves, but unless we address the underlying structure, we are just moving the pieces around. We haven't made any lasting changes just by saying affirmations, or going on a diet, or superficially altering our habits. We've addressed the symptoms without going to the root.

Affirmations change the thoughts but not the thinker. Diets change the eating patterns but not the eater. Willpower holds the negative actions in check for a little while but does not ultimately change the doer. If you only change what you *do,* all you get are temporary alterations to your actions. Shift your *inner viewpoint,* though, and your world transforms.

The physical aspect of power yoga will transform your body—of that there is no doubt. And who doesn't want a more powerful and peaceful body? The real question is do you just want a more powerful and peaceful body, or do you want a more powerful and peaceful life? I will push you, poke you, prod you, challenge you to tap some potential, but ultimately, how far you go is determined by you and your inner viewpoint.

The Western path to "self-improvement" is based on attacking our problems, which we see as the enemy, and ourselves as the victims. We look at the cause, analyze the pattern, and seek out ways to "fix" it.

In the Eastern model, there is no need to improve ourselves, because our real power flows from a force that is in us but not of us. The goal is to simply surrender ourselves and our problems to the highest powers in the universe. The Eastern model tells us not to struggle against our problems but rather to forgive and let go: resist less, struggle less, fight less, and flow more. From birth we are taught to swim upstream, but in yoga practice the goal is to jump into the river of life. Struggle just drains us and fortifies the very thing we want to release.

Surrender is not such a difficult thing once we realize that within us is a brilliance that is already perfect, already wise, already healthy. Problems are just places where we have been separated from our authentic selves. The only solution needed is to become aware of the thoughts and imaginings that are keeping our true selves buried. When you change your focus from limitations to boundless possibilities, from doubt and fear to love and confidence, you open your world in entirely new ways. You stop worrying about fixing what's wrong with you and start living from all that's right within you.

When you focus on the problems, you get more of the same. What you focus on you create. You can analyze the problems, react to them, wrestle with them, take them all personally as though something is wrong with you. But that just keeps the negative merry-go-round circling in your head and leads you to again seek out another plan, another program another 20 percent solution. As Einstein said, "Problems cannot be solved at the same level of awareness that created them."

When you make that deep internal shift from your problem-solving mind to your truth-knowing mind, you don't need to search for the answers anymore. The search for answers is over and the process of more fully accepting and owning what you already know has begun. All that is not authentically "you" falls away, and you have a new center of being that allows you to see very clearly what is needed to effect change in your life. You stop trying to *fix* yourself and start *being* yourself.

It sounds like I'm promising miracles, but this is all entirely possible, and entirely within your reach. Rewiring your mind from within is where it all begins. The actual psychic surgery happens through surrender to a willingness to see things in a new way. It's time to step out of the mental box we keep ourselves in; to turn our worldview upside down and see from a whole new vantage point. When we relinquish the negative beliefs and thought systems based on fear, fight, and limitation, then we open the door to spontaneous and healing insights fueled by love.

The Power of Yoga to Rewire Our Minds

A lot of people think yoga is good for the mind because it reduces stress. But stress management doesn't interest me. Coping is not what this is all about. That's just putting a lid on a boiling brew of poison. I'm interested in *total life transformation,* in transcending stress altogether. I can't change the factors that cause the stress—there isn't much I can do about traffic, or your rela-

tionships, or your job, or your kids, or whatever else stresses you out. But I can show you how to remold your mind and your *reaction* to and *perception* of these things. That is where the stress lies. It's about rising above your reactions and starting to live your life authentically rather than in reaction to everything. When you learn to make this internal shift, you start living from a deeper, more peaceful place. You wake up to your true nature, and suddenly the whole world opens up to you.

There is a story of the spiritual teacher Osho who lived in India and guided many on their spiritual path. One day, a high-ranking Indian politician came to Osho complaining that he was unable to sleep. It seemed no matter what this politician tried, he would toss and turn and rarely catch more than a few hours sleep each night. He was exhausted and desperate, so he went to see Osho begging for guidance on how to relax so he could sleep.

"I'm sorry," Osho told him. "I can't help you. But there is another spiritual teacher down the road who can. Go to him and tell him I sent you, and that you need to learn ways to fall asleep."

The politician was overjoyed and headed off down the road to the other spiritual teacher's home. Several weeks later, he returned to thank Osho.

"Osho, thank you so very much! The teacher taught me how to meditate so I could fall asleep. Thank you, thank you, thank you!"

"Wonderful," Osho replied. "I am glad

you learned how to fall asleep. Now, when you want to learn how to wake up, come back and see me."

This yoga is the ultimate laboratory for awakening. Your yoga mat is a place to invite in stress and meet it head-on, to rewire your mind on a daily basis. All the ingredients you need are there: the challenges, the resistance, the doubts, the frustrations, the fears, the possibilities. You challenge yourself on a physical level, and the mental resistances rush right up to the surface. At those moments, you have a choice: You can either *break down* or *break through.*

Sometimes playing your edge just means taking a leap of faith. You can give in to the limiting beliefs or fears in your mind that hold you back, or you can reframe your consciousness and say "yes!"— "Yes, I can surrender these thoughts, I can let go, I can give up the fight and just be light." The "yes" moments are the breakthroughs, the exhilarating release into transformation.

Opportunity at the Edge

So where do these opportunities for transformation lie? At the place I call the "edge."

The edge is where we come right up against ourselves and what we can do and be. It is the boundary between where we are and where we grow, the place of comfortable discomfort, where all growing and healing happens. The edge is the point in every pose when you are still within your capacities but are challenging yourself to go just a little bit farther. Stepping up to this edge and daring to leap is how you break through and thus break with old ways of being.

We all have an inner comfort zone. Many people keep their thermostat at the same level: they go to the same places, see the same people, eat the same foods, think the same thoughts, have the same reactions. I've heard it said that we have something like sixty thousand thoughts a day, and 90 percent are the same thoughts we had the day before. Think about it: Only 10 percent of your thoughts today are new! We get stuck in a mental hypnosis and become so conditioned that we don't even realize we have put constraints on ourselves.

In India, the way they train baby elephants not to run off is by tying one of their legs to a sturdy tree. The baby elephant will struggle at first, straining against the rope and trying to escape. Eventually, the baby elephant gives up trying, and at that point the owner unties the rope. For the rest of its life, that elephant will never wander farther than the distance of the original captive rope. They don't ever realize they are free, that they can walk a little farther, or even away from the tree that imprisoned them. It is generally possible for people to get into most of the power yoga poses, but it is only when we are tired and ready to come out of it that the pose really begins for us. You come up against fatigue, resistance, fear—all kinds of head trips. Your instinct may be to flee, to say, "This hurts . . . I can't do it . . . I'm out of here . . ." But that is precisely when you have the chance for a breakthrough. That is the edge. That is the moment of truth, when you can transcend your boundaries and grow.

You know you are on your way when you feel resistance, in whatever form it takes, welling up in you. It is *so* powerful when you really start to get that and begin to view those moments as opportunities for growth rather than signals to quit. These moments are precisely what develops strength and serenity.

Dissolving the Blocks Within

Every one of us has limiting beliefs in our minds that hold us back, most of which we aren't even aware of. These beliefs are so germane to who we are that we rarely even formulate them as conscious thoughts. They fester in our deepest unconscious, invisible to the naked eye but powerful enough to run our lives. They are the thoughts that sabotage us right at the moments of greatest opportunity. They whisper, "You can't . . . Who do you think you are? . . . You don't have what it takes . . ." How or why we developed these psychic patterns isn't really important. It's recognizing and releasing them that matters.

So much of life is about our beliefs (i.e., blocks) about what we can and cannot do, and our subconscious mind brilliantly obliges by manifesting circumstances and conditions that reflect our core beliefs. But when you test and breathe through those boundaries, the blocks start to move and eventually dissolve. Of course, if you choose, you can do a ho-hum practice and steer completely clear of your edge. You might even get a few benefits from that. But if you really want *big* results, play your edge in every pose and I guarantee you'll start to see the changes you want in both your body and your life.

Playing your edge in yoga doesn't always mean "going for it," or pushing yourself to do something that overwhelms you. That's ego stuff and it can lead to injury. We're talking about *peeling* away your layers like the layers of an onion, not ripping them off through force. So many students want to just haul out the machete and slice their onions in half to get to the heart. They want perfection and they want it NOW!

What I'm talking about are subtle shifts—maybe holding a pose for a breath longer than you think you can, or stretching a quarter of an inch farther than you have in the past, or even trying a modified version of a pose that seems challenging. Sometimes your edge is learning to do less, to be more tolerant, more patient, more compassionate toward yourself. Ultimately, your intuition knows what you need. As I've said so many times before, your intuition is always, always right and never, ever wrong.

The danger here is that we listen to our ego's voice that says, "No more . . . I can't . . . back off," when in fact our intuitive voice is saying, "Push to the edge . . . break out of the shell that encloses you . . . cross the threshold." The Eight Principles for Stepping Up to the Edge, which follow, can help you learn to distinguish between those two voices. In the "Daily Power Yoga" section of the book, I will give you guidelines so that you can safely find your edge in each pose. But again, only you can know at what point you've hit it and whether you are willing to go beyond it.

The beautiful thing about this process is that as soon as you move through one edge, a new one is created. There is always a new realm to explore, another edge to play. Each layer is a bundle of old, useless information and energy that needs to be released. Physical, emotional, and spiritual muscles grow and stretch, but then they adapt to a new threshold, and it's time to move the bar yet again. It's a continuous lifelong process of constant growth. I have students who come to my studio or Boot-camps who have been doing yoga for fifteen years or more who still have break-throughs on the mat. As one of them said, "It's not a growth that happens once and then stops. It's a limitless process of break-throughs that has no end."

The edge is as much about your world-view as it is your physical potential. The two are intertwined; the key element of this entire Journey into Power program is simply unrolling your mat, doing the prac-tice, and living the principles. Awakening in one realm feeds the other, and vice versa. You can read and intellectualize the idea of rewiring your mind all you like, but you need to set the process in motion if you want to see results.

The Eight Universal Principles for Stepping Up to the Edge

When I teach, I talk my students through the poses and the process. I push them to their edge, helping them tap a new degree of strength and serenity. I speak to their bodies and their minds, taking them through a practice that is meditation in motion. In this process I share the Univer-sal Principles for Stepping Up to the Edge. At moments of difficulty in poses, the principles will do for your mind what a map does when you are lost on a road. They will guide you, empower you, and encourage you to move through bound-aries that once seemed impenetrable. They can be the light that illuminates your path.

These Universal Principles may not resonate with you until you are ready. Right now they are just words on a page, and that's fine. But then suddenly, when you are at the edge, one of these will click. It's the "aha!" moment when you suddenly understand at a cellular level what I'm talking about. So let these sink into your mind. Then, at the right moment, the one you need will ring in your ears loud and clear, like a penny dropping on a marble floor.

These principles are timeless. They ap-ply whether you are an absolute beginner or someone who has been practicing your whole life. As you grow and your yoga practice evolves, these principles will strike you in whole new ways, with different meanings. They're universal—permanent natural laws that never change, like gravity.

Do these Universal and Timeless Principles work? They have worked for me, and I have witnessed miracles in my students. So just open your mind and suspend your skepticism and watch the magic unfold.

Principle I: We Are Either Now Here or Nowhere

"Now here" or "nowhere." Interesting, isn't it, how the only difference, really, is a little extra space.

All life happens in the present moment. All we really have is the moment that is right here, right now, in front of us. Any moment that happened in the past is a memory, and any moment that will happen in the future is a fantasy. Memories and fantasies can be very nice, but they lead us nowhere except into the past, which no longer exists, or the future, which doesn't exist yet. The past and the future are not places. They are, essentially, nowhere. So you see, you are either *now here* or *nowhere.*

The psychology of growth is being in the process and taking it one moment at a time. Change doesn't usually happen in one fell swoop, unless we're talking about earthquakes or winning the lottery. It happens a little at a time, step by step, breath by breath, moment by moment. A small,

steady drip of water can erode a boulder over the course of many years. When you come into the now, you become present to one moment and make a tiny shift, and then the next, and then the next, and before you know it, you have moved your mountain.

Being nowhere as you practice yoga is one of the surest ways to get hurt. In life, accidents happen when someone is not paying attention. You can drive a car at ninety miles an hour and be fine, and you can also drive a car at ten miles an hour and get into an accident—it all depends on your presence. If your energy is scattered all over the place, it's hard to pay attention to what you're doing. I've seen many injuries happen this way. Just recently a student asked me to guide her into a backbend from a standing position, which requires some experience. She had the strength and flexibility to do it, but she wouldn't stop talking. I gently pulled her back up to standing and said, "Your body is ready, but you are not. Your mind is all over the place, and that's the quickest way to hurt yourself in a backbend."

Coming into your body and paying attention to your breath is the master key to anchoring your mind in the present moment. Your breath is always right there waiting for you, the steady, patient guide that will always lead you straight out of nowhere into the *now.*

Whenever you find yourself struggling, you have drifted off into your head, thinking about the past or worrying about the future—in these moments, re-anchor, re-mind, and remember to keep your eyes on the prize of the present moment. Simply follow your breath right back to the present moment and let go of all that isn't happening right here, right now. Tune into the feeling of your breath coming into your body and the feeling of your breath leaving your body. It's that simple: just breathing and knowing that you are breathing. I don't mean thinking of your breathing, just simply a bare bones mindfulness of the breath moving in and out of your nostrils.

Principle 2: Be in the *Now* and You'll Know How

The answer to "how" is always "be in the now." When you tune into the present moment, you rein your focus back in from the distractions happening around you. When you make this directional shift from paying outward attention to paying inward attention, you can really hear what your body is telling you. Your body communicates with you through a language we all understand. It's called sensation. And as with any good relationship, good listening is needed. Hearing your body's voice brings you right into the here and now. Are you experiencing pain? Are you having trouble maintaining a steady flow of breath (a sign that you have gone too far and you've crossed your edge into overwhelm)? What adjustments do you need in order to make the pose more comfortable for you, to make it work?

When you are in the now, a world of options opens up to you. You have more choices and you can modify, dilute, pull back, or push forward as you need. If you are in the now, you will know exactly how far to go, when to push, and when to surrender. You'll know what you need simply because you are focusing on the tangible reality of each and every second.

Tracy could not hold her balance while doing a Twisting Triangle (page 121). She could get her palm to the floor, but every time she spun her upper arm outward and turned her head, she would lose her balance and fall over. She would fall three or four times in each direction, and so she was naturally frustrated by this pose. I tried to give her some tips on how to modify, or some slight adjustments she could make, but ultimately, I told her, she would need to tune into her own body to know how to do the pose. That was clearly not the answer Tracy was hoping for, and she looked even more frustrated. But she kept coming to class and trying the pose, and one day she just blossomed into it as if she'd been doing Twisting Triangle her whole life. When she came out of the pose, she looked at me with a huge grin and mouthed, "I got it!"

Later Tracy told me it was a simple adjustment of creating more length from fingertip to fingertip that made the difference. The slight shift in weight isn't something I or any other teacher could have told her, because every single body is unique and distributes weight differently.

She just needed to tune in and really hear what her body was telling her she needed to do.

You already have the answer to "how" within you; our bodies are encoded with this innate knowledge. The key to accessing it is by coming into the moment. Each time you think you don't know "how" is a clue that you aren't willing to trust your intuitions—use this question as a tip-off that it's time to tune in and trust the light of your inner knowing.

Principle 3: Growth Is the Most Important Thing There Is

I have come to a point in my life where there is nothing more important to me than my own growth. I have three boys whom I love dearly. They are my greatest joy. Yet my own growth is still more important to me. How can I say that? Because if I don't grow, they suffer. If I don't grow, the people I work with suffer. In a sense, if I don't grow, the world suffers, because we are all interconnected and impact one another in powerful ways.

We have two choices: We grow, or we die. It's that simple. Growth is forward movement; anything else is stagnation or, worse, regression. I would even go so far as to say that growth is the answer to the age-old question of the meaning of life. It's the whole point of our journey: to grow and evolve so we can remove all the parts of ourselves that keep us from living in the light, living from our essence, living as our authentic selves. When you remove the blocks, you create flow in your life and go into new thresholds of personal potential. *That* is the goal, and growth is the only way to get there.

Yoga practice is one of the greatest ways to perpetuate growth in all the areas of your life, beginning with the physical. Yoga pokes and prods at our physical limitations, forcing us to experience boundaries not normally experienced. Maybe you can't initially touch your toes in a forward bend, or perhaps your upper body is not strong enough yet to sustain you in Chaturanga (Low Push-Up position, page 87). When you hit that edge, you are faced with the choice to either move through or flee. The choice is always yours. The great thing about a daily yoga practice is that you offer yourself that choice again and again. Going even a little bit farther past your edge is the essence of growth. Physically, you are training your body to go beyond its threshold, and you are one day able to do more. But the psychological lessons that arise in this dynamic are what really catapult you forward in your life. Oliver Wendell Holmes Jr. once compared a person's mind to wet fabric—once stretched, it dries beyond its original dimensions.

The funny thing about growth is the paradox contained within it. It begins not with momentum, or even willingness. It begins with acceptance. You can only grow beyond where you are if you accept where you are in the first place. You can only begin to stretch your limits if you can see and embrace them. It isn't willpower or anger at your limitations that stretches them. It's acceptance. You can never actually grow past your edge if you can't see it clearly and willingly.

Many new students experience a lot of frustration when they first try to take Eagle pose (page 109), a balancing posture that takes new students a while to get in their bodies. In an intermediate class most students take it effortlessly and with grace. In a beginner's basics class, people are usually flopping all over the place like fish on a dock. I watch them get frustrated and annoyed, and remind them that getting angry at themselves for being where they are serves no purpose other than to fuel their frustration and reinforce their perceived limits. If you fight for your limitations, your only prize is that you get to keep them. Everyone started as a beginner, I tell them, and the people who can now do this pose are the ones who accepted even the little bit they could do and worked from there. Just do what you can, from where you are with whatever level of ability you have. When you quiet down and pay attention on purpose, you can actually see clearly where your edge is and play with it from there. But staying focused on what you can't do prevents you from discovering what you can.

So when you hit your edge in a pose—or in your everyday life—instead of giving in to frustration or whatever other reaction surfaces, focus on your commitment to growth and ask yourself: Where am I now and how can I accept, let go, and grow?

Principle 4: Exceed Yourself to Find Your Exceeding Self

If you do what you've always done, you'll get what you've always gotten. It's that simple. If you really want to grow beyond where you are, to change your habits, your body, your mind, and/or your life, you need to exceed yourself. To find the authentic you buried inside, you need to tread into new territory. The new frontiers are within us; the real stretch is internal. You know what you get from doing things the way you do right now. Your best thinking has gotten you where you are. But do you know what you get if you go just a little bit beyond the usual?

The irony of exceeding yourself is that it usually happens after you've perceived failure. The moment when you believe you have no more energy or capability, when you are certain you have to give up, is when you experience the most profound breakthroughs. In weight training, it is in the last two repetitions after your muscles are fatigued and quaking that new growth happens. That's called adaptation. Those last two reps are when the muscle fibers finally tear microscopically so they can repair and rebuild themselves stronger than before. All the reps up until that point were just preparing you for that moment of perceived failure and opportunity.

In a challenging yoga practice, you do your best poses when you are near exhaustion, because you just don't have the strength to resist change. On a certain level you finally surrender: not to defeat, but to the sustaining power of the universe that propels you forward. In those moments your body is weak, but because your spirit is willing, you venture into new territories of strength, power, and peace.

At one Bootcamp, we were going over the alignment of Crow pose (page 107) and I asked if anyone was having a particularly hard time with it. A woman named Alicia timidly raised her hand, and I invited her to come up to the front so we could try it together. She lined herself up perfectly but was afraid to lift both feet off the floor; she feared tipping forward and landing on her head (a common fear in Crow pose). She kept trying and trying, growing visibly more frustrated with each attempt. She looked up at me with tears in her eyes and said, "I just can't."

Though her words claimed defeat, Alicia's eyes said otherwise. There was a spark of willingness in them. "Yes, you can," I encouraged her. "Let's do it together."

So again Alicia tried, and again she pulled back before getting her second foot off the ground. Still, she was determined, and with tears streaming down her face, she lined herself up one more time. I gently guided her up into the pose and held her steady for a moment or two, then let go. She stayed up! After about ten seconds she came down and the entire room burst into applause. Alicia's face was radiant, and for the rest of that Bootcamp, every time we did the Crow pose, she climbed right up into it and held it with an enormous smile

on her face. She'd broken through and discovered a whole new level of herself.

When you hit your edge in a pose, it's time to ask more of yourself. If you can relax with your edge, you'll realize you are stronger than you think you are. You have more capability than you believe you do. If you just breathe and maintain equanimity in the face of adversity, you can exceed even your biggest dreams for your body and for your life.

Principle 5: In Order to Heal, You Need to Feel

The real irony of spiritual growth is that instead of being some miraculous experience, it feels a lot more like going to pieces. As soon as we open ourselves and our lives up to be healed, suddenly all kinds of unpleasant feelings come to the surface. We experience fear, disappointment, shame, even rage—certainly not the rosy, glowing epiphanies they promised in the brochure!

If you ask for wisdom or higher virtues, know that they only come through trials and tribulations. If you ask for inner peace, God will send you a storm in which to practice and cultivate peace. We get what we want through practice. There's no such thing as a free lunch in the spiritual realm. You can stay stagnant in your comfort zone on or off the mat, but in order to transcend yourself and gain wisdom, you need to go through the fire, walk on hot coals, travel through the desert of your own mind, and come through on the other side transformed.

In order to heal, we first need to feel. We spend our entire lives stuffing down emotional and physical injuries, but these wounds don't really disappear. Cellular memory is a powerful thing, and deep within all of us is a record of every feeling we tried to suppress, every emotional scar we keep buried, every physical ailment we thought was healed. To truly heal from the inside out, this psychic debris must be brought to the surface so it can be released.

The things that come up for you on your yoga mat won't always be easy. As I said, the thing I love about yoga is that whatever is in there, yoga will find it. Physically, old injuries may feel activated, so they can be healed and released. You may feel a strong sensation, a tightness, and even pain as your muscles stretch to dissolve emotional knots and release your body's holding patterns of tension. New aches and pains may arise as your body shakes off however many years of stress and toxins. You feel the truth of your lifestyle in your body. It's right there. Your thoughts, your reactions, your emotional patterns—they're right there in your body. So as you come into all of these different postures, they are just tools for exploration, and then opportunity for release.

Emotional pains may surface as well, because our bodies store the energetic remnants of these emotions deep within the tissue. Backbends symbolize fear of looking into the past, so a Camel pose (page 131) may trigger a buried painful memory or traumatic experience from many years ago. Our hips are emotional storage houses, so hip openers like Pigeon may release angers you weren't even aware you had. Chest-opening poses like the Wheel (page 134) may stimulate buried sorrows or flood you with love and appreciation for someone in your life. Though your instinct may be to stuff these all back down, they are coming up now, so that you can feel them one last time and finally release them and be free. And ultimately, being free from your excess "stuff" is what this is all about. As Kahlil Gibran said, "The pain you feel is the breaking of the shell that encloses you."

If you are really willing to feel, you can create real changes in your life. On the other side of these pains of purification is true peace. There is a famous story about Renoir and Matisse, who were friends. One day, Matisse visited his friend Renoir and watched him paint. Renoir suffered from terrible arthritis, and every stroke of the brush caused him immense pain.

"Why do you do this to yourself?" Matisse asked.

"Because when the pain disappears, the beauty remains," Renoir replied.

Thankfully, most of our pains will pass. There is a yogic principle that promises everything is fleeting—nothing is permanent, not even pain. The road to enlightenment always passes through confusion, frustration, and pain. People sabotage their practice—and their growth—because they give up in those difficult moments. But if you stay in it, stay open, relax, and breathe, a breakthrough is *right there* on the other side. Every problem has a solution, and staying in our calm center allows us to receive it.

We can be light, even in the face of adversity and pain. If you can say, "I'll laugh about this in five years," why not laugh about it now? If you think it's hard to open up, to let go, to quiet down, to feel, to bring levity to moments of adversity, to practice yoga, try living your whole life without these things!

Principle 6: Think Less, Be More

I can always tell when students who come to my classes have been trained in Iyengar (a style of yoga developed by B. K. S. Iyengar that focuses almost entirely on perfect alignment). They do beautifully refined poses, with every muscle and joint in the right place, but they never look like they are having any fun. Don't get me wrong, I think Iyengar is an excellent basis for learning alignment and I have a lot of respect for his method. My only complaint is that these students never seem to come out of their heads. They know all the mechanics but don't have the flow that comes from getting out of your head and into your body. I always tell Iyengar students who come to my classes or Bootcamps, "You've been learning to tune your violin beautifully; now I'm going to teach you how to play music!"

Once you learn the mechanics of a pose—what goes where, what rotates which way, and so on—the only thing left is to get your brain out of the way and just relax into it. You can psych yourself in or out of anything, not to mention think a pose to death. Analysis paralysis is the ego's way of keeping you rooted in your intellect rather than your spirit. But when you drop your brain, you actually give your body and soul a chance to shine.

Aerodynamically, a bumblebee should not be able to fly. But bumblebees don't know that, so they just do it. They open their wings and take off, oblivious to the fact that their round little bodies weren't designed for flight. Wouldn't it be great if we were all like bumblebees, unaffected by beliefs in our limitations?

The key to learning yoga poses is to take your brain out of it. You can line it up, take my cues, and do whatever you need to make the pose feel comfortable, and then from there, just let go and glow! See if you can perform with half your brain tied behind your back. Come out of your thoughts—your doubts of "I can't do that," your worries of "Am I doing this pose right?," your fears of "Am I going to fall?," your frustrations of "Why can't I do this as well as she can?," and your ego resistance of "If I can't do this perfectly then I won't do it at all"—and just be in your body.

When you let go mentally, there is a shift physically. Doubt your doubts and they vanish. Feel your fears and they fade. Let go of your worries and they fail to materialize. What will it take for us to really get it that life is about letting go?

My friend Krishna Das, a kirtan (chanting) master, said the most important muscle to cultivate is the "letting go muscle." It is the hardest one to locate but the one most essential to develop for true inner peace and physical radiance.

Just think less, and be more. Let go and let good flow in. Let go and then you grow in so many wonderful ways that your brain doesn't even know about yet. That's the beauty—that there is a supportive force in the universe there to protect you if you stop trying to control it all and just let it in.

Principle 7: We Are the Sum Total of Our Reactions

There is a story of a Chinese farmer whose wild stallion ran off one day. All the neighbors gathered around, clucking their tongues and saying, "Very bad luck!"

"Bad luck, good luck," said the Chinese farmer. "Who knows?"

A few days later the stallion returned with a whole herd of wild horses. The farmer corralled all the horses, and all the neighbors gathered around and said, "Very good luck!"

"Bad luck, good luck," said the farmer. "Who knows?"

A week later the farmer's son was trying to break in one of the wild horses. He got thrown off the horse and broke his leg. All the neighbors came around and said, "Very bad luck!"

"Bad luck, good luck, who knows?" came the reply.

Several weeks later the Chinese army came marching through the village looking for able-bodied youth to join the army and fight. When they came marching into the farmer's house and saw that his son had a broken leg, they left him alone and moved on.

"Very good luck!" said all the neighbors.

"Bad luck, good luck, who knows?"

That's technically the end of the story, but it could go on and on. Does it ever actually stop? Isn't that all of our stories in one way or another?

We don't really have experiences in life. What we have are reactions to experiences. Things don't happen to us. Things happen in and of themselves, and what we do is react to them. It's not the existence of standstill traffic that affects us, because if it's happening, say, across town and we don't know about it, it doesn't bother us. But if the cars are at a dead stop on the very road that we need to take, suddenly we are activated, and we react to the existence of traffic. It's not the traffic that we are experiencing. It's our reaction to it.

Built into our hardwiring as humans is the fight-or-flight response, which we needed way back in the cavemen era to keep us safe. But we've evolved, and though the threat of predators is minimal, the response system remains strong. When stress happens, the fight-or-flight mechanism is activated, and we instinctively gear up to do battle or flee the scene. This holds true whether we are faced with a major crisis, like being attacked by a mountain lion, or a much smaller stress, like a spat with a clerk, spouse, or stranger. Of course, there are varying degrees, but the brain interprets all stressful events the same way and triggers the automatic response.

But there is a third option, which is neither fight nor flee, and that is to just *stay and breathe.* If you start to see the reaction rising and feel your emotional feathers getting ruffled, just step back from yourself, come back into your body, watch your breath, and feel the reactiveness dissipate. If reactions happen, let them go, come out of your head, and anchor into your body.

I'm not talking about becoming a zombie. The goal here is not to become emotionally neutered. What I'm talking about is finding a way out of getting hooked into an automatic response because of your reactiveness. Halting your cycle of reactiveness allows you to have a perspective shift, so that you have the chance to respond in better, more positive ways. With a perspective shift, a forty-five-minute traffic jam can suddenly become forty-five minutes of alone time to sing out loud at the top of your lungs, or meditate, or do whatever your daily routine doesn't afford you the time to do.

Yoga practice gives you the opportunity to create a gap between stimulus and response that gets wider and wider, and in that gap you have the option of choice to change your response, rather than zooming into autopilot. A world of different ways to handle things opens up to you. Suddenly you can read into situations in-

stead of just launching into action or reaction (which is really just an automatic repetition of an old action). This is how we ultimately learn to manage and transform our emotional states, and how stress can make us better rather than bitter.

There will be poses that feel uncomfortable to hold at first. If your hips are tight, for example, holding a Warrior I or Warrior II pose for a while may be difficult. You haven't stretched and strengthened those muscles yet, so they start burning almost right away. Your immediate reaction will probably be to get out of the pose . . . fast! In that moment, you have a choice. You can go along with the automatic reaction and response and come out of the pose. Or you can remember that every pose begins precisely at the point when you want to come out of it, widen the gap, breathe through your reaction, and stay. A little burning in the muscles never killed anyone. The worst that can happen is that you end up with a well-toned body and a deep sense of accomplishment.

We react thousands of times every day, usually without our conscious awareness. As if by reflex, we get annoyed when the train is delayed, or discouraged when our boss reprimands us, or angry when our kids misbehave. We instinctively launch into anger and fear, but these reactions keep us trapped in unconscious behavior. When we start to open our eyes to our patterns of reaction in our yoga practice, however, it helps us to learn to recognize and slow the reactiveness cycles in our everyday lives. Working your edge teaches you to rise above the stress you feel and move into equanimity. When you do that, you are operating from your center, from cause rather than effect. You don't have less stress from doing yoga; you just learn tools to rise above it.

Perhaps the greatest example of nonre-activeness in our time is Gandhi. During the most controversial stage of his protests, Gandhi was approached by an English official who told Gandhi he was very sorry, but that he had to arrest him. With complete calm and certainty, Gandhi replied that he was not sorry at all.

They locked him up, yet he did not react with anger or indignation. When people asked how he could remain so calm, he said it was because he would not allow anyone to walk through his mind with their dirty feet. He believed that other people's actions belonged to them, not him. He stayed his course, focused on his goals, and did not let himself get hooked by reactions that could have derailed him. As a result, he ultimately changed not only his own experience, but the entire world's.

Principle 8: Don't Try Hard; Try Easy

Trying hard invites strain and struggle. Trying easy gives you the levity and freedom to fly. When you try hard, you are using willpower. But willpower never works and will always fail you. That is because willpower is based on brute force as opposed to soul force. Brute force is like trying to lift a Chevy truck with your bare

hands. Soul force is having a pulley to raise it right up. Willpower comes from your intellect, but soul force is powered by your connection to the infinite universe. Your muscles can help you move heavy furniture, but your soul can help you move the earth. There is a power in the universe more powerful than you are, and all you need to do to access it is *relax, breathe, and surrender.* The Latin root of universe is "uni," which means "one," and "verse," which means "passage." One passage: I take that to mean that each of us has our own authentic path. We just need to stop trying, stop willing, and just let it happen. The easiest place to see this distinction between brute force and soul force is in your life's work. If you love what you do, if it is a natural extension of who and what you are and makes your heart sing, then even the most extreme efforts will have lightness to them. The universe works in tandem with you and it all flows. For me, teaching yoga isn't a job so much as what I was born to do, so I don't hold it as a chore. If, however, you are not aligned with your work—if it doesn't reflect your authentic self—suddenly everything feels like a task. Everything is too hard, too much effort, too draining. *True* success seems miles away.

What does it mean to "try easy" in yoga? It means that you go from seeking a better pose to just being in it. It's a deep sense of letting go—not of the effort, but of the struggle. Postures can be achieved through struggle, but the struggle itself limits both your immediate opening and how far you ultimately grow in yoga. Struggle creates tension in your muscles, which constricts you, and in your mind, which limits you. If you relax and stop resisting and reacting, you'll just know what you need to do in the pose.

Trying easy is a state of mind that enables you to go into the fire, but also to discover the calm, cool center within it. Physical intensity is, of course, key when it comes to going to the next level, but within that is a release. The Buddha said, "Make yourself light." He didn't say to make yourself heavy, or to fight. Take your poses seriously, but take yourself lightly. Smile to yourself; laugh inside.

A student named John who comes to my studio had been struggling with Dancer's Pose (page 116) for some time. He would fall out of the pose almost immediately every time. I watched him get more and more frustrated every day, and whenever I said, "Okay, let's take Dancer's Pose," he would get that hard, serious look on his face. Then he'd get all tense and lose his balance within seconds of taking the pose.

One morning, when we got to Dancer's Pose and John was engaged in his usual struggle, I walked past his mat and quietly said to him, "Don't try so hard. Just let go and see what happens." John looked skeptical, but then he shrugged and said, "Why not?"

John reached back, took hold of his foot, and gracefully arched forward into a beautiful Dancer's Pose. I stayed behind him and reminded him not to tense, not to fight, just to breathe and trust his body and his ability. He held the pose for the full five breaths and came out of it slowly and deliberately, rather than in his usual method of falling. The huge grin on his face said it all.

When you find that you are straining, whether in a yoga pose or in life, you're probably trying too hard. Your ego is in it, and you are driven by an ambition that ultimately creates imbalance and suffering. That is the point when you should ask yourself: Where am I holding on? Am I holding on to tension, or to my ideal of what I am "supposed to" be doing? Where can I let go more? Where can I struggle less? Where can I just surrender?

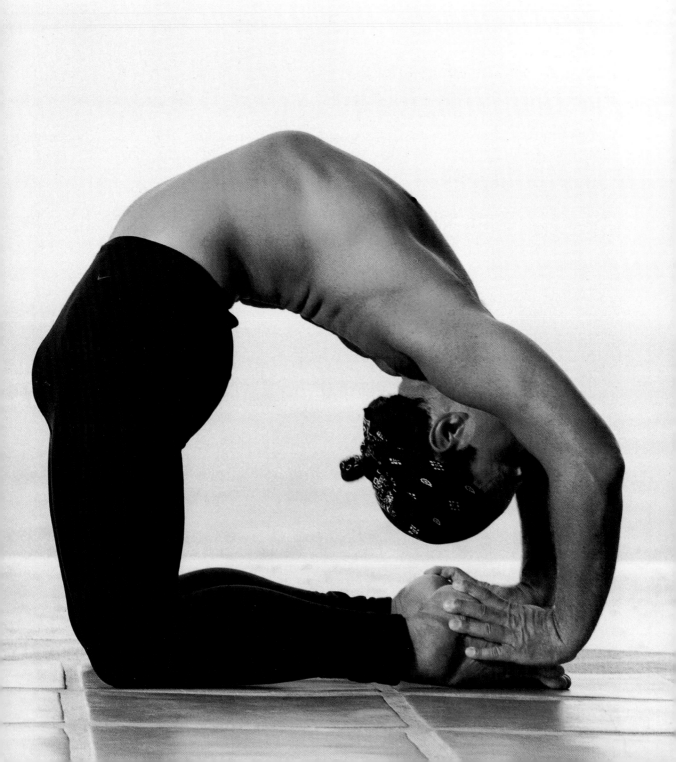

I know of no more encouraging fact than the
unquestionable ability of man to elevate his life by
conscious endeavor.

—Henry David Thoreau

PART 2

Daily Power

Yoga Practice

PEOPLE OFTEN ASK ME HOW I CAME TO DEVELOP BAPTISTE POWER VINYASA YOGA. I NEVER REALLY "DEVELOPED" IT; IT WAS MORE AN EVOLUTION, A NATURAL PROGRES-

sion of studying, researching, practicing, teaching, and just living my life. For many years I was a student of the traditional forms—Iyengar, Ashtanga, Bikram, Krishnamacharya, Raja yoga. I've also studied traditional forms of fitness, martial arts, and have trained hundreds of professional athletes for peak performance. Over the years, I combined what I thought was the best of the best from the East and West and left out everything else. I wove it all together into one powerful, all-inclusive practice.

My style of yoga is called Baptiste Power Vinyasa Yoga, "power yoga" for short. It is just what the name implies: vig-

orous and powerful. Strength is a pillar of my style. The word *vinyasa* means "flow," or the linking of one movement into the next, one breath into the next, the presence of mind from one moment to the next, and that is another pillar. When you combine these factors along with heat, you get what I believe is one of the most dynamic, life-changing forms of physical and spiritual fitness. It is the perfect blend of sweat and serenity.

If I had to describe Baptiste Power Vinyasa Yoga in two words, I would call it free style. It contains fifty-three poses (or "asanas") that are linked together by connective momentum. I'm not attached to any one tradition that sets any rigid rules. I have come to understand that there is a perfect process for each individual, no matter what age, weight, or fitness level, and honoring that is more important than adhering to one narrow and rigid path. I follow the natural laws of the body, which dictate balance and counterbalance, control and surrender, pose and repose, modification and acceleration. You will get all the benefits of the more traditional methods while still leaving room for creativity and fun.

What Power Yoga Is *Not*

Power yoga is different from most typical forms of yoga. We don't try to bend you into a pretzel or force you to chant. I'm less interested in burning incense than in burning away the excess baggage that weighs down your mind and body.

I know from my experience that many people are intimidated by yoga, and I think the traditional yoga world does a lot to perpetuate that. I have spent my whole life researching and refining a style of yoga that is real-life practical without losing the essence of yoga's transformational power. You don't need to be open-minded to do my style of yoga. You just need to *do* it; the results will speak for themselves.

My style of yoga is not just for those seeking cosmic consciousness. I've taught all types, from politicians to professional football players. The people who come to my Bootcamps and studios range from Harvard MBAs and stay-at-home moms to celebrities and rock stars. Power yoga is for everyone, whatever they are seeking. It's my mission to bring this five-thousand-year-old practice down off the mountain and make it accessible to anyone, from any background, looking for total physical, mental, and emotional transformation. A lot of people assume yoga is gentle and passive, and definitely not a workout that creates physical transformation. But this is anything but sedate. Power Yoga is a dynamic, energizing form of exercise that sculpts, hones, and tones every muscle in the body. It will kick your butt, but no matter what physical shape you are in or what limitations you believe you have, you can definitely do this! It is purposefully challenging and active so that it can catapult you from wherever you are right now to whole new thresholds of physical and mental power.

You don't need to be some super-flexible version of Gumby in order to do power yoga. Any dimwit can wrap their legs around their head; it has nothing to do with health. There is a lot of showmanship that goes on in the yoga world, in which people get hung up on displaying how much they can contort their bodies. But there is no research that shows that wrapping your legs behind your head will give you better health, and frankly, I don't think it will make you a better person. There is no proven health benefit to being overly flexible. In fact, hyperflexibility can be a sign of weakness. Over time it can lead to overstretched ligaments and tendons, which create imbalance and instability in the body.

I don't care about contortions. My focus is on creating real-life flexible strength, stabilization, and full-body integration. There is nothing wrong with taking pride in your body and what it can do—a little vanity can even be healthy. Where I make the distinction is between practicing for the sake of ego and self-image and practicing for inspiration and practical usefulness.

I'm not a guru, nor do I want to be. I don't believe you need to follow a guru to do yoga "right." Yoga is a path that is shared by many, but each person experiences his or her own growth in his or her own way. I want to give you the tools to learn to follow your own wisdom, your own intuition, your own heart. I want you ultimately to be your own teacher, to have a connection and a perception about your own body and what's right for you. Yoga is about discovering *your* essential and authentic self, not someone else's. Everyone can do power yoga. *Everyone.* No matter what level of fitness you are, how much you weigh, or what your genetic makeup may be, you can do this. Everybody is different, and every pose can be made to fit every body. As I have said thousands of times to students, you just start where you are with whatever level of ability you have, and from there, the sky's the limit. Strength and suppleness come with time, as long as the spirit of willingness is there.

Why Power Yoga Works

I love power yoga because it works magic. But you don't need to take my word for it—in fact, please don't! You can easily prove to yourself how effective power yoga is in creating transformation. The best way to demonstrate the value of something—anything—is to see it work for yourself.

Power yoga works for so many reasons. It works because it is simple and right in line with how your body is designed to move and operate. It builds functional intrinsic strength rather than superficial strength. It empowers you to purposefully use and train your body the way you do in real life—bending, stretching, lifting, reaching, twisting—so you can move through your everyday motions with more ease, more agility, more power, more grace. How often do you use the motion of a bicep curl or a boxing kick in your everyday life?

In traditional fitness we tend to break up the components of strength, flexibility, stamina, and cardiovascular training into their own levels of importance based on our goals, and put relaxation, meditation, and our psychology in some other category with the stuff in our lives that we would do if we had time. I liken this approach to baking a cake: You have all the ingredients you need—flour, sugar, eggs, milk, and so on—yet you never mix them. If you were a guest at my home I wouldn't serve you just a cup of flour! In power yoga we blend all the key ingredients into what I call global training, which means to train the whole person. It embodies strength, flexibility, stabilization, stamina, cardio, and mind power all in one session.

The health benefits are multilayered, going beyond just the external. All the internal bodily systems are activated and improved as well. Your nervous system is soothed or energized as needed (through deep rhythmic breathing); your glandular system is balanced, creating hormonal harmony (from inversions); your cardiovascular and circulatory systems are invigorated (as a result of the flow); your digestive and metabolic systems are stimulated (from the heat of the ignited fire within); and your elimination system is activated and regulated (from sweating and from the movement of lymph, the body's sewage system). Every single cell in your body benefits.

Power yoga works for so many people where other fitness and therapeutic methods have failed because the results from yoga are immediate, fueling your motivation to continue. You don't need to wait weeks before seeing and feeling positive results. From your very first practice session, you experience shifts energetically, muscularly, mentally, and emotionally. Your muscles tingle from head to toe, your blood is flowing, your mind is clear, your

spirit is revived, you are full of stamina and breath; you feel *alive!* Once you get even the smallest taste of these results, you have all the motivation you need to keep going.

Power yoga is effective on deeper levels because it gives you a new awareness of your body. It brings breath and consciousness to all your muscles and tissue and you really make the connection between your mind and body. From there, you start to get more in tune with what your body needs, on and off your mat. You start to make new habits, and then those habits make you! You begin to see that your body requires your love, compassion, attention, and care. Whenever you give anything positive attention—a flower, a child, your body—it blossoms.

Sometimes waking up to your body can be like waking up in the middle of the night with your house on fire. You suddenly see the danger all around you: all the damage you do to yourself, the conditions your lifestyle has created, all the negative energy that is weighing you down, all the unkind and unhealthy ways you treat your body. Once you awaken to the truth of what's happening inside you, it is not so easy to go back to sleep. You naturally and easily start making choices that cleanse, heal, and free your body and soul.

The Pillars of Power Yoga

There are five foundational pillars of my power yoga: breath, heat, flow, gaze, and the abdominal lock. All are essential pieces of a dynamic and healthy power yoga practice. Each one of these enables you to have the deepest experience every time you get on your mat. When integrated together, they launch you into new dimensions.

Breath

Your breath is the key to unlocking your body's potential. Maintaining steady, rhythmic breathing is the *single most important element* of yoga practice. Your breath is what links your mind to your body, and you to the present moment. As you become skillful at matching your breath to your movements, the two will no longer feel separate, but rather one thread that carries you through the fabric of your practice.

Your breath is pure, raw energy that sweeps through you like a cleansing wind. It carries prana, or life force, to every molecule in your being. With every inhalation you literally bring new life into your body, with every exhalation you clean house.

Through matching and mirroring your movements with your breath, you peel away the layers of resistance. Your breath is what sustains you at your edge and allows you to move past it into new mental, emotional, and physical frontiers. In this way you are meeting inner resistance with a neutralizing force. If you can stay calm and breathe through your pose, that layer of resistance dissolves.

The breath we use for asana practice is called *ujjayi breathing* (ooh-jy-yee). The ujjayi breath is an audible breath that has a soothing, rhythmic, oceanic quality. It is done by contracting the whispering muscles in your throat to create a long, hairline thin breath. You do not breathe all the way down into your abdomen, but rather into your chest, lungs, and back. In fact, if you breathe into your belly, your power is lost.

Here is a step-by-step breakdown of how to do it:

1. Bring your first or second finger to the soft spot between your collarbones.
2. With your mouth closed, breathe in through your nose, feeling the gentle retraction of those muscles beneath your finger. It should feel as though you are whispering in reverse. You are closing the airways a little, so it's kind of like breathing through a straw. Imagine the breath as a cleansing wind sweeping right in through that soft spot at the base of your throat.
3. For the exhalation, put your hand in front of your face as if it's a mirror. Gently retract your belly and, with your mouth closed and the muscles in your throat still contracted, exhale through your nose as if you were going to fog up that mirror. The exhalation is exaggerated and extended. It is important to keep your mouth closed or you will lose energy on the exhalation.

This is the ujjayi breath. In, out, in, out . . . deep and free, rhythmic and steady. The volume of your breath both on the inhale and the exhale should be equal to each other. In general, you inhale as you reach up and open in poses, and exhale as you fold down or close.

If you're getting dizzy, you're probably forcing it too much. Just relax and let it be effortless—not taking in too much or too little air. It's like a woodburning stove: too much oxygen and you burn up the fuel too quickly, not enough and the fire goes out. A steady flow keeps the internal flame burning.

Throughout your practice, keep remembering to *breathe . . . deep and free!*

Heat

If you try to reshape cold glass, it will shatter. Heat it and you can form it, bend it, and shape it any way you want. Your body is just the same: Heat it and it becomes pliable. Muscular motion creates heat that softens your tissue and makes you malleable.

The strong flow of power yoga fuels the inner furnace, and the breath fans that fire throughout your practice. The combination of motion and breath builds what I call healing heat—the kind of heat that melts away tension and accomplishes decades of growth and release within days. Tension, after all, is just stuck energy, and when you start the internal heat moving, all that does not belong gets burned away. All the resistance is consumed by the intensity of your internal flame.

A hot room can boost the purifying fire, so at my studios we heat the room to 90 degrees to help students build and maintain a liquid quality to their move-

ments. The heat also helps you sweat. Sweating is one of the most important mechanisms of natural healing, since it enables the body to release toxins, metabolic debris, and excess fluids. It also gives the liver and kidneys some much-needed rest, because their usual burden of detoxifying and purifying the blood is lessened. The skin is the largest elimination organ of the human body, and the more you sweat, the more toxins you release. Besides, it feels so good to just let the sweat pour out of you!

American Indians consider purification of the body inseparable from purification of the spirit. They have used the sweat lodge as a powerful process of physical and spiritual regeneration for thousands of years. I have experienced firsthand the transformative power of this ritual. A Great Lakota elder leads our Bootcamp participants through a powerful prayer sweat in the mountains of Montana, during which many of them receive profound insights and have life-changing experiences.

At first you may not like the heat. It may feel uncomfortable. But pretty soon the purifying power of it hits you. It feels so good, you wonder how you could ever practice without it. When I do workshops at places where I cannot heat the room, longtime students who are used to the heat always remark that their movements are so much less fluid in the cold room. They feel stiffer and less able to move deeply into the poses. They suddenly realize how the heat softens their muscles and how much more they get out of the practice that way. The heat heals; the heat protects your body from injuries; the heat sets you free.

When you do your practice at home, try to do it in the warmest room you have. Of course, it's ideal if you have a room in which you can raise the temperature, but if you can't, at least turn off the air conditioner or close the windows. Maintain the flow of the practice to sustain your inner heat, which will help avoid injury and allow you to go further into your poses.

Flow

In my style of power yoga, each pose flows right into the next. You are synergistically taking your body through multiple motions, angles, and planes, and channeling all of your energy into one synchronized symphony. It is a beautiful melding of fluid and flexible strength, mental focus, deep breathing, and stability in motion.

Flow is the absence of resistance. When you bring flow into your practice, you let go into the movements and create a liquid quality that inspires deep release. It allows you to build magnificent momentum and heat and move through your practice in an effortless, seamless manner. Flow encourages meditation in motion: When you ride the flow like a wave, it moves you out of your head and into your body and the present moment.

On the most basic level, flow creates dynamic energy that keeps your internal heat up and your heart pumping steadily.

This brings the cardiovascular element into your practice, which facilitates weight loss and an overall increase in health.

Drishti

Drishti means "gaze." In yoga practice, it means fusing your eyes to one point. This focus sends soothing messages to the nervous system and brings the mind from distraction to direction. The eyes are the lens of the mind, and with drishti you are focusing your consciousness. Drishti allows you to slow your mind and engage more deeply in your practice.

It's very simple to do: At the beginning of every pose, relax your eyes and set them on a fixed point. It can be anything—a spot on your mat or the wall. Your eyes should be soft and tender. Hold your gaze steady for the duration of the pose. That's all there is to it.

Part of drishti is samadhi, which embodies "neutral vision." *Sama* means "even" or "neutral," *dhi* means "vision" or "seeing." Neutral vision means to see without judgment, without ego, without impatience. Samadhi is to see through a clear lens, rather than viewing your experience through the rearview mirror of your past perceptions. Cultivating samadhi on your mat will help you bring that quality of mind into your everyday life.

Drishti is key to all balancing poses. Balance comes from a calm, nonreactive mind, and I always remind my students that we set our mind beginning with our eyes. If our gaze is steady and focused, our mind will be, too, and we can better maintain our equanimity. Wandering eyes equal a wandering mind; focused eyes equal a focused mind.

Uddiyana: Core Stabilization

In every pose, we activate what is called the uddiyana bandha, or "upward lifting lock." A "bandha" is a lock that anchors you into your stability and strength. This bandha is a static muscular contraction used to focus attention, stimulate heat, and control the life force within us. Uddiyana is a gentle lifting of the pit of the abdomen toward the spine. Through uddiyana, you draw attention to the core of your body, the epicenter of all movements. Making this core the focal point causes you to move, breathe, and have your being from your center. Thus grounded, your body roots and can then lift into a state of weightlessness.

Uddiyana tones the internal organs and also plays a vital role in protecting your lower back. By drawing your belly into your spine, you stabilize and support your lower back and torso in your poses. In the bigger picture, a lot of people experience dramatic relief from chronic back pain by building this core strength and removing the stress on their lower back. A strong core—your torso, which includes your back and abdominal muscles—is the foundation to true, real-life body strength. In the same way that a chain is only as strong as its weakest link, you are only as strong as your core. In this practice we focus on building core power and torso stability, and uddiyana is a master key.

Uddiyana is simple in explanation but takes some exploration to understand. Basically, you contract your belly and lift it up gently toward your spine. As you draw the navel inward, the abdominal muscles follow, creating a hollowness under the rib cage and driving the breath into the upper torso and chest. Remember, you will be engaging uddiyana in every pose, hence the need to be gentle so that you can maintain it throughout your entire practice.

Why Daily?

When I first opened my studio in Cambridge, we put up signs that said, "For good results, three times a week. For life-changing results, five to six." If you want decent results, three times a week will do. But if you're really looking to transform your body, your spirit, and your life, do power yoga every day—you'll be amazed by what happens.

A regular practice keeps us on track. Practicing daily is a way to check in with your body on a consistent basis. Your body communicates in the language of sensation; listen to it. What is your body feeling today? Where are you stiff, tense, stuck . . . and what does that mean? Are you off-balance? Do you feel strong or drained? Is your breathing smooth and free or ragged and congested? As the connection between your body and mind becomes clearer, you start to really see what's going on for you each day, and you see how your habits or actions manifest in your system.

When you get on your mat, the results of how you treated your body the previous day are right there for you to witness. Your mat is a mirror; when you step onto it, your actions are reflected back at you. You directly experience cause and effect, both good and bad. You feel how heavy food creates heavy energy, and eating lightly creates vitality. Maybe you feel the effects of that second glass of wine, the chocolate bar, or your third cup of coffee, and realize that you don't really need it. Or maybe you start to see how many hours of sleep you must have to be able to function at optimum levels. All the feedback you need about your body's requirements and tolerances becomes available to you. Never again will you have to turn to "experts" to know what you need. You are cultivating an awareness of your own well-being, learning to listen to your body and honor your intuition.

Practicing three times a week helps, but you live your life all the time, so why get your energy flowing only three out of seven days? You can't really awaken if you only plug in three times a week. Since yoga creates new wiring in you, it's much harder to start and stop because you lose the momentum and the cumulative effects of practicing consistently. Yoga is all about moving energy, and when you don't do it, the energy becomes stagnated. You then have to expend more energy to get it moving again. It's like a car: You use less fuel if you keep it running than if you turn the ignition on and off. The more you practice, the easier the asanas become and the more benefits you get. You get longer, stronger, and more supple every time you get on your mat, and eventually, you astound yourself and flow right into poses that once seemed impossible. It's a simple but crucial rule that for any level of transformational success you must develop the spirit of repetition and consistency. Repetition is the mother of skill, and skill is the mother of mastery.

Even if you are a beginner, I recommend doing power yoga daily. It's not like other forms of exercise, so there is no danger of overtraining as long as your practice is balanced. The more you do, the better you'll look and feel, the stronger you'll become, and the brighter you'll shine.

How Long Should I Practice Each Day?

It's better to do a little bit of yoga a lot than a lot of yoga once in a while. So rather than doing two hours once a week, you'd be better off doing twenty minutes every day. Ideally, you should do an hour and a half of power yoga each day, but if that's not possible, do whatever you can. Some days I'll do a long hour and a half practice in the morning; other days I'll do forty-five minutes in the morning and forty-five minutes late in the day. Sometimes I'll just do twenty minutes in the morning.

The practice session outlined in this book is the equivalent of a ninety-minute class. At the end of this section, I have also given you a formula to help you tailor your daily practice to fit into your schedule. It's important that you follow one of these programs rather than skipping around and designing a session on your own. Nothing about the power yoga routines is haphazard; the sequence of postures is laid out in such a way so that each posture prepares you for the one that follows. Jumping right into the backbending series, for example (which comes sequentially toward the end of the practice), could have the unfortunate effect of shocking a muscle, pulling a ligament, or straining a joint.

The best time of day to practice is first thing each morning before doing anything else. It will prepare you, center you, and give you fortitude and clarity for the day. If mornings are not possible, choose a time of day when your office or home is as quiet as possible and free from distraction. That's important. If evening is best, then do it at a reasonable hour rather than after the late news. The tired mind does not absorb well, and the tired body does not move well. In addition, you tend to be less aware late at night, and injury could result. You want sufficient energy—both mental and physical—sustaining you when practicing these postures.

Find the timing and pattern that works for you, but I encourage you to get on your mat at least once a day even in the beginning, even if it's just for twenty minutes.

Consistency is the key to sparking power in your practice. Then, as you get more in tune with your body, you'll know how often and how much you need.

Building Healthy Poses— The Master Principles of Alignment

The Pillars of Power Yoga—breath, heat, flow, drishti, uddiyana—give you the tools to create a graceful and strong practice that integrates the whole body and the mind. You will use all of these foundations to build a healthy practice, and you specifically want your individual poses to be sound. The building blocks of safe poses are what I call the Master Principles of Alignment.

The Master Principles of Alignment help with the how-to element of your practice. It's the "what goes where, what rotates which way, which muscles and joints do what" part. Your poses don't need to be perfect, but they do need to be healthy, and these principles will help you understand the mechanics of what you are striving for when you get on your mat.

The Master Principles of Alignment bring you back to your natural and ideal alignment, which over the course of your life, due to various stresses (like the pull of gravity), has been thrown out of balance. By incorporating these principles into your practice, you will learn how to master the biomechanics of healthy movement.

Eventually you won't need to focus individually on these principles because they will become a part of you and your unconscious competence. Just as in mastering a musical instrument, where you spend hours practicing scales and chords, over time they become second nature and just flow out of you naturally, creatively, and spontaneously.

Principle I: Build Your House on a Rock

The New Testament says a foolish man builds his house on sand. If you build it on sand, it cannot withstand the weathers of life: hurricanes, storms—even the slightest breeze could cause it to crumble. If you build your house on sand, it will wash away at the first sign of turmoil. The same is true for your body in yoga postures.

Building your asanas on a rock means first creating a strong physical foundation. The foundation of almost every pose is the base, the part of your body that is rooted to the earth. Whatever is touching your mat is your foundation. In standing poses, your feet are the foundation. In inversions, the palms of your hands, your shoulders, your forearms, or the top of your head are the foundation. If you are lying on the mat, your back or belly is the foundation.

Once you have a stable foundation, you can begin to work the rest of the pose, from the ground up. If you build a pose on shaky footing, there is a good chance you will lose your balance and find the pose frustrating. If you take the time to get really secure and stable in your foundation, however, you set yourself up for success.

Power in all standing poses comes from the feet. It's drawn up through the legs, triggered through the hips, and projected out through the torso into the arms and hands. In a standing pose, take the time to feel your feet firmly planted to establish rapport with the floor. Then go deep into your legs, feel your strength, square your hips, elongate your torso as life goes up and awakens your arms and fingers. For inversions, like Shoulder Stand (page 142), it's the opposite: stabilize your shoulders and upper arms on the ground, then align your chest, hips, and legs. If you fall out of a pose, don't race back into it haphazardly. Start over from the foundation and take the time to rebuild it from there.

The width of your foundation (the space between your feet) plays a role in the stability of standing poses. The wider your base, the more you are able to activate spinal extension, but you lose general stability. If you feel unbalanced in a standing pose, shorten your stance. Eventually, as you develop more strength, you can widen your base.

Principle 2: Establish Neutral Alignment

Neutral alignment involves bringing your body into a balanced relationship to gravity. It is, in essence, the ideal of each pose: a natural, stable posture in which you create even lines in your body.

If your car is out of alignment, you can still drive it, but eventually the tires wear unevenly, putting stress on other parts of the vehicle. It becomes an accident waiting to happen. The human body is the same. If your hips are uneven or a knee is collapsing in or splaying out, the entire structure is unstable, thus creating imbalances, aches, and pains throughout the entire body, potentially leading to long-term damage. Yoga practice is repetitive training, so keep in mind that repetition of your movements can result in either mastery or misery.

Neutral and symmetrical alignment of all body parts is the first element of injury-free movement. The whole is the goal, and the integration of each piece to the other—legs, pelvis, torso, arms, head, and neck—creates a foundation of true power and stability from which all the poses begin and end. When you integrate the various parts of your body in neutral alignment, you create a sense of naturalness in poses. You fight less and breathe more. You don't struggle to stay in balance or to hold the pose. You line up the energy patterns in your body properly, and suddenly you achieve a weightless state. You feel free, tall, uninhibited.

You'll know when you've achieved neutral alignment in a pose when suddenly it ceases to be a struggle. You fall into a perfect relationship with gravity and you feel a sense of strength, stability, and overall balance. In that moment, you make the pose yours. Every body is different; no two people have the exact same formula to reach neutral alignment in any pose. The tips and cues I will give you for each posture will help lead you toward this, but

you'll need to play with your alignment to find what gets you there.

This yoga practice will teach you to notice the imbalances, the postural habits, the compensations, and the negative physical adaptations that have developed over your lifetime. After all, you are a walking auto-biography. If you have spent your whole life drawing your shoulders up to your ears, or tilting your pelvis a certain way, or caving your chest in, over time you'll become aware of these unconscious holding patterns. The daily repetition and systematic diversity of the poses in this practice allows you to scan your entire body. You will see that one side of your body is stronger than the other. The strong side is tighter, the weaker side more flexible. One side can do more, one side can do less.

When you see these imbalances, be compassionate with yourself. It has taken you a lifetime to accumulate them, but with daily power yoga practice it will take far less time to neutralize them. The postures demand that you work equally on the right and left sides of the body, the front and the back sides of the body, the lower and upper parts of the body, and here is where the corrective element comes into play. The postures give you the opportunity to draft the ideal blueprint of a balanced and coordinated body.

Principle 3: Stack Your Joints

Though stacking your joints is part of what is needed to achieve neutral alignment, it is not all that goes into it, which is why I teach it as a separate principle. Stacking your joints means lining up your joints along one track, as in "ankles in line with the knees, which are in line with the hips." The three weakest links in the human body are the knees, the lower back, and the neck, and protecting those in your yoga practice is essential to avoiding injury or long-term damage. Stacking your joints in line and creating right angles keeps all the hinges going in the direction they were meant to go and protects the joints, ligaments, and tendons.

An example of stacking your joints is in Warrior II pose (page 94), in which it is imperative that your knee is stacked directly above your ankle, making your shinbone and thigh into a perfect right angle. This protects the knee from strain. Your shoulders should be stacked directly above your hips, so that your spine is one straight, neutral line. This keeps your pelvis and core centered.

Almost every posture requires that you stack your joints in some way, and I'll show you how to do it for each one so that your poses are healthy and aligned.

Principle 4: Balance, Control, and Surrender

There are strength and surrender elements in every posture. We always hold one part of the body strong, which allows another part of the body to release. Certain muscles are held firm, and others relax into the pose. Some muscles are supporting and some are supported. This balance between the two actions is what makes yoga such a unique and powerful form of fitness: It accentuates strength and grace, stability and flexibility, hard and soft, so that your entire body is engaged in a balanced way. In yoga we say we use everything but overuse nothing.

You may feel strong in one pose while others feel impossible. Since yoga exposes weaknesses, you can't just muscle through the practice. If you have strong, bulging biceps, they will only get you so far. It is not about developing one set of muscles in your body, but rather about developing your entire body and remembering that many parts make up the whole. Everything—cells, muscles, joints, and spirit—works together to provide support as well as exert strength, whether they are leading or following. This is how your whole body comes into balance and every muscle is ultimately engaged and toned.

Balancing control and surrender is central to *traction* within poses. When anchoring one part of the body and pulling through another, you create a natural length, space, and extension. For instance, in Bow pose (page 129), the legs resist and are active and the spine and torso are passive (lower body controls, upper body surrenders). The legs work strength, the spine works length. This creates space between the vertebrae and a natural traction through the torso.

Ultimately, yoga is about creating space: space within your spine; space within those secret pockets of tightness; space between your muscle fibers, bones, and joints; space between your doubts and beliefs; space between your emotions and reactions; and most important, space between your ears. With new space we become an open vessel to receive new insights and inspiration.

I'll tell you which muscles to control and which ones to surrender in each pose, but as you start a regular practice, you'll just start to know. Your body is already wired to understand this, so over time it will just come naturally to you.

Principle 5: Work from the Bones

When you move with consciousness from your bones, all the muscles, tendons, ligaments, organs, and connective tissue will naturally follow. "Bones leading, muscles following" is a good mantra to remember.

What does it mean to work from the bones? It means moving from deep within each body part, stretching as though you were pulling yourself apart at the seams. If I told you to lift your arm, chances are you would raise it automatically and not think much about it. But if I tell you to raise your arm leading with the bones, it feels different, doesn't it? It's deeper, more powerful, and ultimately more graceful when you use your internal infrastructure rather than mindlessly flapping your limbs around.

Working from the bones is the key to all the rotations we do within poses. Most poses contain some element of rotation, for example: in Downward Facing Dog (page 76), you spread your shoulder blades away from each other and then slide them down your back; in Warrior II (page 94), you rotate both thighbones outward from the hip socket—the right one goes clockwise, the left one counterclockwise; in Namaste Forward Bend (page 125), you rotate both thighbones counterclockwise (if your left leg is forward)—this naturally helps you turn your hips like a steering wheel to center your pelvis.

This may all sound a bit complicated at first, but don't worry, it's really not. It will all come naturally once you get flowing. For each pose, I'll highlight clearly the alignment principles that are in effect, so you'll know all the subtle techniques to focus on.

Coming Out of a Pose

Out of the corner of my eye I was watching Bob take the Wheel pose (page 134). I knew he'd been struggling with this, so I was happy to see him let go of his resistance and press up into a full backbend. The muscles in his arms and shoulders were quaking from the effort, but he held it for the full five breaths. When it was time to come out of the pose, he just collapsed down onto his mat. I was certain he had jammed his neck. How could he not, crashing down on the crown of his head like that? Bob was lucky and didn't injure himself that time, but I reminded him and the rest of the class that any fool can get into a pose, but only a wise person can come out of it with conscious grace.

Never, ever snap-release out of a pose! The most common way people injure themselves in yoga practice is when they are coming out of poses. They think, "Great . . . I'm done . . . let me out . . . ," then twist and yank their bodies out of the pose they were holding rather than easing out. The momentary relief you feel from quickly releasing a difficult pose isn't worth anything if you wrench your neck, or your knee, or your lower back.

Vinyasa flow is an unbroken stream in which one movement leads into the next, breath leads into breath, pose leads into pose, transition leads into transition. The poses between poses are poses! Take your time to ease back out of a pose the same way you got into it. Do the exact steps you took in reverse, working from the top down to your foundation. Injuries can come in any physical activity, but many of those sustained in yoga practice can be avoided if you pay attention and transition with awareness.

The Seven Most Common Mental Mistakes in Yoga Practice— and How to Avoid Them

Almost every person new to yoga practice is subject to seven major mental mistakes. I'm including myself here. When I was a beginner I made most of these mistakes, too. Sometimes I still make them, but many years of experience have taught me to recognize when I have done so. With time, you'll be able to see these patterns in yourself and get back on track more quickly.

As a teacher, I am here to help correct these errors—gradually and sometimes immediately—in order to help you improve your awareness and overcome these pitfalls on your path to mind/body mastery. Eliminating just one or two of these seven common mental errors can catapult your yoga practice and your life beyond what you thought or allowed yourself to think was possible. Eliminate all of them and anything and everything is possible.

Mistake 1: Believing Your Doubts

No matter who you are, I promise that you can do more than you think you can do— not because you were born double-jointed, or because you were blessed with strong and pliable muscles, but because when you believe you can, you've already moved half the mountain. Everyone has the capability to shine. *Everyone!* All it requires is an unbending faith in yourself. Just start where you are and do what you can do, and there will be no stopping you.

Believing your doubts is one of the most insidious mind tricks that your ego can play on you. Doubts are not real; they are just illusions created to keep ourselves from taking risks because we are so afraid of failing. Your yoga practice will reveal the real limits that you confront in your body, but it may astound you to discover that many of the limitations you perceive as physical are actually mental. When you believe that you can't, you can't. I see this form of self-sabotage almost every day in my classes.

There was a woman at one Bootcamp who refused to try Tree pose (page 117). It is relatively simple, but it does require balance (which comes from the mind). She insisted she would fall if she lifted one foot off the ground. She was frozen. I offered to assist her, but she refused. I never push anyone if they aren't ready, so I just let her be, but the other participants tried to help her.

"Just try it," someone said. "It's really not hard, I swear."

Nope. She wouldn't budge.

"It's all mind, really," another said. "You just think you'll fall, but you won't."

No amount of convincing worked. She wouldn't lift that foot for anything, completely convinced she would topple over if she did. When we came out of Tree pose, she went right on with her practice along with the rest of us, but to my mind, something was lost. She'd hit the edge of how far she believed she could go and backed away from an opportunity to grow. She let her doubt take over and never gave herself a chance.

We are like clay. We can reshape ourselves and transform if we are willing to. There's nothing static here. We may believe our limitations and tell ourselves that "this is just how I am," but that's not true. As the saying goes, fight for your limitations and the prize is that you get to keep them. We have the capacity to move beyond where we are right now. All we need to do is have faith.

Faith comes from knowing that there is so much more beyond just you. There is an unlimited power that wants to come up and surface in your body and your life right now. When you say yes to it, it can flow through you and take you into realms you may have thought impossible to reach.

Just doubt your doubts—that is true faith.

Mistake 2: Despising the Days of Small Beginnings

There is a verse in the Old Testament that asks, "For who hath despised the day of small things?" Any creative person knows not to despise the days of small beginnings—the first brushstroke, the first word on a blank sheet of paper, the first note played. Those fragile beginnings are precious, for no masterpiece could ever come into being without them.

In all of life, yoga practice included, there are sequential stages of growth and development. A child learns first to roll over, then sit up, then crawl, and eventually walk and run. Each step is important and each one takes time. No one step can be skipped. If you observe the first three years of a human being's life, you can see it truly defines the days of small beginnings. Those first wobbly steps lay an essential foundation.

Occasionally a person will come into my class not knowing a thing about yoga and yet three months later look as if she's been doing it for years, simply because she didn't expect perfection. For her, yoga is a joy to discover and she takes it one day at a time. On the other hand, there are people who come to a yoga class once but never return. They arrive with their achievement brains in full force and effect, and when met with imbalance, awkwardness, or weakness in their bodies, they experience frustration, embarrassment, fear, and doubt. They are driven by the unconscious attitude that if they can't do it perfectly, they won't do it at all.

The fact is, an open-minded beginning yoga student is like an infant learning to take his first steps. You won't see him give up just because he lands on his butt a few dozen times! On a ten-point scale, if you are at level two coming into class or starting your own practice at home, and you desire to move to level eight, you must first go through levels three, four, five, six, and seven. The edge you'll hit can only be moved through if you stop hating the fact that you are a beginner at every new step and start embracing it.

The awkwardness and fear in the early days of your practice will fade soon enough, and you'll forget very quickly the things you weren't able to do. It's a funny thing about yoga; over time you tend to forget the physical struggles you experienced along the way. So do not despise the days of small beginnings, for it is in those moments that you open new doors to discovery through which all things are possible.

Mistake 3: Embracing Tradition Over Intuition

No one person can tell you what is right for you. Not in a pose, not in a diet, not in your life. Every single body is unique, and only you can ever really know what is right for you. You can hear advice, seek out guidance, and even ask for help, but ultimately, it is you and you alone who knows what is best for you.

Enlightenment about your body, your mind, and your life is a very individual process. Teaching becomes problematic when we prescribe that there is only one way of doing something. It is said that the path to enlightenment is like a bird flying in the sky: It leaves no footprints behind. That is why traditions that claim theirs is the only way are absurd. Tradition is valuable for what it can teach us, but the minute it becomes absolute, it negates the most precious human resource there is: our intuition.

One of the singular appeals of yoga is that it promises a definite technique by which we can make ourselves independent of preceptors, teachers, or gurus. But so often we are not shown that side of yoga in the West. We are given teachers, or "gurus," who establish themselves as divine intermediaries and claim to hold in their hands the key to our enlightenment. Traditional yoga often sends students the message that they must follow teachers or tradition to the letter, that they know nothing in comparison to the guru, that it's the teacher's way or the highway. Believe me, I've been around the yoga world my whole life, and I've seen every angle of intimidation, humiliation, and blind devotion. Since I was a boy, I have witnessed many soul-searching people get swallowed up into the unthinking atmosphere that surrounds popular gurus. To this day, I'm stunned to see educated men and women blindly following a master. Regardless of what inconsistencies arise, they make excuses for the master, as though they have forfeited their powers of discernment and common sense.

Many gurus control their followers through the brilliant process of contradiction. Do what they say, and they promise you will achieve enlightenment. The catch is that the tasks or problems they present you with are altogether unsolvable. You become emotionally and spiritually absorbed in the problem, then are taught that you need the guru to guide you through such a big and confusing process. You doubt yourself and come to rely more on the guru, believing that he is the one with the answers.

At one point in time, my life was guided in this fashion. I could not break away, because at that time I believed my guru possessed the only key to personal power. Whatever he said was right. If I didn't understand something, it was because of some defect in me, not the master.

I did the long hours of meditation, chores, asana practice, and endless study, all with small amounts of sleep. I was the true brainwashed yogi disciple.

Eventually, I woke up and saw that I was only regurgitating what my teachers had told me. Without personal common sense and intuition, I realized, self-actualization was impossible. I could never really find the wisdom in myself if I only listened to what others were telling me.

I later came to realize that the stakes in this kind of game are very high, and that people will do things in that state of mind they would normally not do: bending their bodies into positions that are ridiculous for their body type; memorizing sutras until their heads spin; or following diets, rules, vows, and techniques that make absolutely zero sense for who they are.

If I sound a bit critical of gurus, I should clarify that the target of my criticism is the ignorance, hypocrisy, and downright spiritual dishonesty of many who profess to be gurus and masters in this ancient practice. The honest teachers are the ones who are willing to kick themselves off the pedestal and be real.

People bow to an orange-robed master, and then find out one day he's not wearing any underwear. He may have amazing and wonderful things to teach us. But when you start thinking of him as holier than thou, you are falling into a trap. My father told me, "Don't be so fast to trust, but don't automatically distrust," and I think that's the best advice anyone can give.

Your intuition is always right. ALWAYS. It is never wrong. And it is important that we get that. To the degree that I remember that, and listen to my intuition, my life flows and abundance pours in: the right people, the right guidance, the right circumstances. But when I ignore my intuition, I create a mess.

The question is, when are you going to start trusting your intuitive power?

Here on your yoga mat, start practicing intuition in action. Don't follow me, or anyone else; follow yourself. If I tell you to do something and it doesn't work for you, question it, modify it, play with it to make it work for you. I will push you, poke you, prod you, guide you, but it's up to you to tune in and flow from what's right for you.

Mistake 4: Not Recognizing That the Prize Is in the Process

There are no prizes for perfect poses, no ultimate goal here. Yoga practice is a journey with no end. You'll grow and even transform along the way, but ultimately there is no arriving. When that moment of revelation hits you, it is one of the most important internal shifts. A sincere yoga practice is just that: a *practice*. It's a daily practice to help you gain a completely different and improved perception of everything within and around you. This kind of transformation requires a radical surrender and a radical commitment to the process of growth. There is a reason this book is called *Journey* into Power; it's not Arriving into Power!

I remember realizing early on that there were no limits as to how far I could go in a pose; I knew I'd never get bored, because there was always another depth to reach. So perhaps I got into it initially because of the challenge. But I stayed with yoga and made it my focus because of the beauty of the process that yoga continues to take me through. One of the reasons I teach yoga is that I want to share in that shift from being goal-oriented to being process-oriented. The more I teach, the more I learn that both teaching and learning are an unending process of refinement.

There are two basic mind-sets. One involves viewing a posture as something to be achieved, a goal to complete; how far you get in the posture is what counts in your mind. This is a typical mistake many beginners or Type A personalities make, and it often leads to frustration or injury. Focusing on a goal means trying to get your body to do something you want it to do, rather than surrendering to the process. Because we are so focused on performing, we potentially miss out on something magnificent.

The other mind-set views the posture as a tool to explore and open the body. Instead of using the body to get an ego boost, you use the posture to get to know and gain understanding of your body and mental patterns. The poses then become experiments to reveal and work through the resistances that block you, so you can ultimately move through them. Approaching the postures as goals makes you less sensitive to the messages your body is sending you.

It is so common at first to push too hard and fast instead of allowing the body to open at its own pace. It is always best to trust the natural order of things—the progressive development through time. A rose has timing. So do trees, and seasons. Only humans are in a hurry. If you try to open a rose before its time of blossoming, you break off the petals. So, too, if you rush your own unfolding you will cause greater harm than good.

Once you've been doing your practice for a while, you'll probably notice that it has cycles. You're into it, then out of it, then into it again, and so on. Even now, after practicing seriously for over twenty years, I go through these cycles. And if you're like me, the challenge comes when you start to plateau. I have discovered that yoga is the art of dealing with plateaus. Part of the process is sometimes taking three steps back in order to go six steps forward and vice versa. Sometimes you'll even feel as if your practice is getting worse, but really that is all part of getting better. Sometimes you feel as if you are completely stuck, and then suddenly it seems as though a door opens and you break through.

In China, farmers begin the process of growing bamboo by burying the root four feet under the earth. For a couple of years they water it, fertilize it, and nurture it without seeing it or even knowing if it's still alive. Then suddenly, after two years

of patience and love, it shoots ninety feet into the sky within sixty days!

The point is that sometimes results are barely visible, but every fraction of an inch of progress is meaningful. Don't seek better poses, a perfect body, or immediate inner peace. Let go of the ambition and embrace the practice of peeling back your layers. Just be where you are, play your edge, and the prizes will be revealed along the way. Transformation is an endless process to be lived. It cannot be captured or possessed; you can only participate in it.

Mistake 5: Falling into the Trap of Competition and Comparison

Yoga is usually presented as being non-competitive. At its heart that is true, but your ego may pull you into the trap of trying to keep up with the proverbial Joneses. So just in case you didn't know, let me tell you: The Joneses are very messed-up people!

It is very common to start feeling competitive as you come to your mat. You look around the class and see someone in a fierce-looking Warrior pose and judge your pose pathetic in comparison. Or maybe you're struggling with Downward Facing Dog while your friend holds it effortlessly. But if you watch two dogs stretching, you won't see them peeking over at each other to see who's doing it better! The action is instinctual, natural, and without ego.

In a yoga class, you may view the strengths of others as proof of how weak you are, and spend your time feeling sorry for yourself, making excuses for yourself, beating yourself up, and using this to confirm your self-doubts. Or worse, you ignore your real weaknesses and push yourself to catch up with people who are "better" than you. You only feel good as long as you keep up or, better yet, outdo.

Or maybe your ujjayi breathing is deep and rhythmic in comparison to the person next to you, who sounds like a lion with asthma. Perhaps you can go into a full Wheel pose and your friend needs to take the modified version. Instead of paying attention to where you are in your process, you focus on people who are worse off than you, making you feel superior.

Competition is identity-based, but the real path to power is spiritually based. As you get more experienced in your practice, you must look more deeply into your competitive instinct, for if you don't explore it, it will continue to rise up automatically and unconsciously. It takes you over without you noticing it, and the next thing you know, all you can focus on is how much "better" or "worse" you are than those around you. You've lost sight of what really matters.

What's needed is an understanding and appreciation for where you are. When you are secure in yourself, you can appreciate the strengths and successes of others without feeling challenged or threatened by them. You can even learn from them.

Comparison in and of itself isn't a bad thing. Comparison is a basic mode of thought, the very notion of which is wrapped around progress. How can you know how far you've come if you don't compare it to where you've been? How can you gain insight on ways to improve and grow without learning the difference between you and those around you? Competition is right if it feeds your soul and growth; it's harmful if you use it to put you above or beneath others.

Don't be intimidated by other people's pretty poses, or gloat in feelings of superiority when those around you are struggling. Just watch the feelings of competition and comparison as they come up, then detach and let them go. Don't feed them by fighting them. Don't get caught up in struggling with them. Don't kick yourself for feeling them. And don't deny them. Just accept, appreciate, relax, breathe, and focus on peace. That's the way to grow out of unhealthy comparison in yoga . . . and in life.

Mistake 6: Not Recognizing That Sometimes Less Is More

In yoga practice, sometimes less is more. Not always—sometimes more is still more—but there are moments to push and moments to surrender. You learn to distinguish by trusting yourself and honestly gauging where you are and what is needed. You can struggle to get into the ideal of a pose, but you may gain more by lessening, backing off, or modifying the posture. It takes a long time for ambitious overachievers to get this concept, especially if they are accustomed to succeeding in life through hard work. They excel because of intellect, daring, effort, and guts, and suddenly they unroll their yoga mats and discover all these qualities actually impede their progress. For these people, less is usually more, and their wiring prevents them from accepting that as anything but weakness.

The root of all misery is attachment. We are obsessed and attached to our outer appearances and physical capabilities. We have an image of ourselves, and when we can't maintain it, our identity as we know it begins to crumble. Power yoga tends to challenge that image, forcing one to experience unexpected limitations and boundaries. That coming apart, of course, is the breakdown that precedes a breakthrough.

Karen was a typical Type A personality when she started coming to my classes. At thirty-five she was a vice president at a large international bank, and by outward appearances in excellent physical shape. She loved what power yoga was doing for her body and thrived on the challenge, but still struggled with certain poses. Karen's nemesis was Revolving Crescent Lunge (page 98). Every time she tried the pose, she would lose her balance and fall out of it. She knew the modification was to drop her back knee, but to Karen, modifying meant defeat. Intellectually, she could hear me saying that there was a pose for every body and that everyone should do what they can, but her deeper mental wiring dictated that that didn't apply to her. The pose was hard for her because her hamstrings were tight from years of running, and eventually, as you might have already guessed, Karen pushed it too far and hurt herself.

If you recognize yourself in this description (in any way!), less may be more for you. The edge for you to learn from might not be how far you can go in a pose, but rather what you need to do in order to make your pose healthy. Remember, there is no such thing as a perfect pose per se, only perfect presence and equanimity. In yoga we make inner peace our only goal and the rest of the benefits just kind of happen along the way. By searching for equanimity rather than perfection, we lay the foundation for emotional stability no matter what happens.

How do you know if less is more for you? First and most obviously, if you are injured. If you have a chronic problem like a bad shoulder or knee, you'll need to take care not to aggravate it. Yoga isn't about barreling through pain, but finding modifications so you can work with and through it. Will, who has been coming to my studio in Cambridge ever since the day it opened, has a bad shoulder from an injury that occurred years ago. He comes to practice five days a week and simply does what he can while still protecting his shoulder. Some days he does only two Sun Salutations instead of six, or he drops his knees in Downward Facing Dog, and some days he just does the poses that engage only the lower body and stands in Ragdoll (page 78) while we do the others. He's not doing a "perfect" practice, but he is certainly doing a more authentic one than some of the people around him, who are huffing and puffing and straining past their edge.

Experiencing what I call "bad pain" on any level is another signal that less is more. There is a difference between "good pain" and "bad pain," and making that distinction can mean the difference between gently moving the boundary of your edge and pushing yourself to injury. Bad pain will be clear to you. It is usually sharp and electric; the message your body is sending you is a deep "uh-oh . . . back off." It's crucial that you obey your body in those moments. Physical pain is real feedback—it's a warning sign that could mean you're going too far. Ignoring genuine pain almost certainly invites injury. Good pain, on the other hand, feels more like a deep sensation in your muscles. Good pain might be soreness, or a deep stretch, or intense holding in a pose. It's that place of comfortable discomfort.

Last, you'll know it's time to pull back a little if you start to panic in a pose. If you cannot maintain equanimity and steady, rhythmic breathing, it is a signal that you are going into overwhelm. When you panic, you lose your ability to intuit your body, and you move into survival mode, in which your only focus is making it to the end. As soon as this happens, *you know you've gone into your head!* Slam on your mental brakes, relax, and come into your body, into your breath, and into the present moment. Observe your body's reactions and sensations to find the edge between comfortable discomfort and overwhelm. The key to mastering that edge is to keep your breathing deep and free and to maintain serenity during strong sensations.

If you are fearful in a posture, it's wise not to try to override it in order to be courageous. You have nothing to prove to yourself or anyone else, and pushing yourself to that extreme negates what you are trying to do in your practice. You want to exceed yourself, not damage yourself.

By the way, Karen did eventually come back to her yoga practice, but she was in many ways a different person as a result of her injury. She saw how pushing herself relentlessly could cause her not only physical injury on the mat, but emotional damage in her everyday life. She admits that she is a work in progress; every day she now tries to live the lesson of "less is more" in one way or another.

Mistake 7: Not Understanding Your Resistance

Along with any growth process comes resistance. The two are as intertwined as the moon and the tides.

As a person who has been involved with yoga and personal growth for years, I wish I could tell you that I have conquered resistance. But I have not. Sometimes I still have to drag myself to my mat. The first five minutes are pure resistance, but then it starts to melt and I get into the flow. Ironically, the days that start with the most resistance usually turn out to be the best practices.

Resistance can be a great teacher. It exposes your state of mind and being—your fears, attachments, and limiting beliefs. Then it's up to you to choose whether to continue protecting your existing patterns or to expose them to the light.

The postures are designed to open up and reveal every pocket of resistance in the body. They give us the opportunity to dissolve this resistance and break through to the other side. Facing the resistance without fighting it is the only way to grow out of it. Ignoring your resistance ensures you'll stay stuck in it. You can try as hard as you like and find ways to move around the blocks in your path, but the thing that blocks your path *is* your path. The resistance that surfaces is the next place you need to look, the next edge you need to play.

We all know that the mind and body affect each other. Emotional tensions live in the musculature (your muscles and joints can actually hold on to memories of past trauma and tension) and through years of accumulated tensions and dis-ease, the body becomes a storage house for unconscious holding patterns.

Have you ever noticed the posture of someone who is really depressed and down? His chest caves in, his shoulders slump downward, and his head falls forward. His physical body actually starts to mold itself around his heartaches. His compressed chest protects him by literally making it harder to experience and express deep-seated emotions. If he were to do a chest-opening pose like Camel (page 131), the force of the emotions that might come from opening his chest could make him uncomfortable.

He then has a choice. He can either start complaining about what an uncomfortable form of exercise yoga is and vow never to do it again, or he can look objectively at his resistance, stay with the pose, and observe what emotions it brings up. If he chooses to remain closed off, what will limit his ability to move to the next level is not his body but rather his fear of seeing the truth that can set him free. If he sticks with it, though, he'll become aware of how the opening of his body is facilitating an opening of his mind. His mental resistance will subside and his posture will change.

The key to working through your resistance is always a radical inner surrender, a calm determination, and a commitment to letting go!

In yoga, you encounter all kinds of resistance—resistance in the tissue, resistance in the mind, resistance to doing your daily yoga, and resistance to changing the habits and lifestyles that impede growth. Anytime you feel stuck, look for what it is that is blocking you—your blind spots— and the path you need to take will reveal itself.

Getting Started

It's time to unroll your mat and begin! This is where your Journey into Power goes from concept to reality. We can talk about it, explain it, dissect it, and debate potential mistakes you may make, but it all comes down to unrolling your mat and just *doing it.*

What to Expect

If you are a beginner to this style of practice, you may feel awkward and frustrated at first. But I assure you, nearly everyone starts this way. Just remember that *all* our bodies are meant for yoga! Make it your own.

The spirit of flexibility gives you physical malleability; the attitude of strength gives you real muscle. I have watched three-hundred-pound people come to my class as beginners and tap into their personal power and unique process of transformation simply because the spirit of willingness was there. I've had guys walk into class with bulging muscles from weight training and within a few poses their arms are shaking. Eventually they thrive on the flexible strength that comes from using your own body weight as resistance, but they need to experience their own evolutionary process like everyone else. Be gentle and patient with yourself, and you will be great.

The beginning will be challenging, but beginnings usually are. Once you get going though, it gets easier and will start to come together in an effortless series of breaththroughs.

You'll experience ups and downs and the inevitable plateaus as you go through your practice. Each day will be unique. Sometimes the energy and drive is there, other times it's a struggle. Your body is just like your mind in that it has moods. The moment you step onto your mat you'll know the mood. Work with it. After all these years of practicing I still have days where I'm right on, and other days where I'm struggling. Some days your practice will flow like a clear, cascading river; other days it will feel like swimming through glue. Just do it anyway! Modify, dilute, and discover what modifications you need in order to make the poses healthy and workable for you, but don't overreact and give up. Remember, breakthroughs come at the moments of perceived failure. If your ego says no, let your spirit say yes! Willingness, repetition, and consistency will lay the groundwork for true transformation.

You might be sore after your first practices. This is completely normal—you're conditioning deep muscles. You may even discover muscles you didn't know you had! I actually love the feeling of being sore, because soreness is heightened awareness and a part of positive change. If you are really sore, keep practicing. A good hot practice will wring out the metabolic acids and flush your muscles with fresh nutrient- and oxygen-rich blood, and the ache of soreness will disappear.

When we do our Bootcamps in Mexico

or Hawaii, I encourage students to float in the seawater as much as possible. The saltwater is rich with minerals that draw the toxins out of the muscles. If you don't live near the sea, you can try adding natural mineral salts to a hot bath to get the same effect. If you have the time and resources to get a massage, I recommend that as well; it will help drain the lymph and metabolic debris from your tissue.

Random aches and pains that have plagued you may vanish, but new ones may surface to be healed. A very fulfilling aspect of teaching yoga is hearing the unending number of students who tell me how longtime aches, pains, and ailments had suddenly disappeared after only a few practice sessions. Just recently, a student told me about a neck injury she had sustained years ago. She had suffered residual pain and stiffness that prevented her from being able to turn her head all the way to the right. After a month of practicing power yoga, she regained full mobility in her neck. She laughingly credits power yoga for giving her the entire right side of her world back.

Your longtime back problem may disappear, but you may now experience other small healing crises, like soreness in your hamstrings. This is all natural; these new aches and pains are a part of the healing and strengthening process. Your body is going through a metamorphosis, a deep and true reconstruction. You may at times even feel as if you're getting worse before getting better. Sometimes healing,

strengthening, and opening in one area exposes a hidden weakness in another. Don't worry; just relax and stay the course.

Intense emotions may surface when you first start your practice. They can come out of nowhere and hit you with depth and intensity. This is also natural. Let them come up (and maybe even have a healthy gut-level cry if you need to), and just allow that energy to move through you so you can release it. Don't react; just relax and sit with it. Keep breathing and know that maybe, for the first time in your life, you are cleaning house and waking up.

What You Will Need

The one thing you must have to begin is a yoga mat. A mat prevents slipping and provides a little padding. You can find yoga mats at almost any sporting goods store, a yoga studio that sells equipment, or on-line. The kind I recommend is a thin, nonslip, washable mat that I import from Germany. I sell these mats (along with other yoga supplies) on my website, www.baronbaptiste.com. Many students keep a towel spread over their mats to prevent their sweaty hands and feet from slipping. Props like yoga blocks, blankets, and straps can help you modify poses in your beginning stages.

The Postures

Congratulations! You are about to take the powerful stride toward mastery in body and soul! What follows are the fifty-three postures that will comprise a well-rounded and dynamic power yoga practice, all in ninety minutes. The poses are grouped into eleven series, each with a distinct purpose that plays a potent role in the overall practice. For example, the first series, Integration, brings you into your body, into your breath, and into the present moment. The third, the Warrior Series, creates vitality and energizes your whole body; later in the practice, the Inversion Series creates hormonal harmony and brings everything back into balance.

The eleven series are:

1. Integration Series: Presence
2. Sun Salutations: Awakening
3. Warrior Series: Vitality
4. Balance Series: Equanimity
5. Triangle Series: Grounding
6. Backbending Series: Igniting
7. Abdominal Series: Stability
8. Inversion Series: Rejuvenation
9. Hip Series: Opening
10. Forward Bending Series: Release
11. Surrender to Gravity Series: Deep Rest

For each pose I give detailed instructions on how to get into it, the corresponding breath, alignment tips, and the vinyasa to connect you to the next pose, just as if I were teaching a live class. As it applies to each pose, I'll include the external and internal benefits, the risk factors to watch out for, modifications to make if you are a beginner or have an injury, and a spiritual focus to weave into your practice. Every pose is accompanied by a photograph so you can see the ideal to work toward. Some have additional photos showing modifications that can make it easier or more challenging as needed. My goal is to demystify this process and make it work for you in your life, right now, so the more you know, the healthier and more powerful your practice will be for both your body and soul.

As mentioned earlier, the series are done in a specific order that is designed to work globally and systematically through all the dimensions of the body. At the end of this section I will show you how to create practices that can fit into your schedule. I will give you the formula to use to create a healthy and effective practice if you have only fifteen minutes, half an hour, or an hour, so you can fit a practice in every day.

1. Integration Series: Presence

The Integration Series is where it all begins. This is where you step out of the world and into yourself, where you come out of your head and into your body. Here you activate your ujjayi breathing, the deep life-changing breath that will unite your mind and body and ignite your internal fire throughout your entire practice.

The Integration poses bring you into the present moment, quieting the everyday chatter of your mind and focusing your energy toward rejuvenating, rinsing, and healing. Here is where you get calm and come to center, establishing your rapport with the floor and getting a sense of your body's mood in the moment. You set your intention and put a prayer to your practice. It all starts here, with these three initial poses that unite your body, breath, and mind.

The moment you step onto your mat, make a commitment to shelve the problems and worries of your life. Just put them on ice for now; you can pick them up again later, when you're done, if you're really attached to them. Our goal, of course, is to have you *let go* of all the useless baggage and energy you bring with you to your mat, to shift you into a different space, so that when you return to your everyday life you have a whole new perspective. You can look at the same issues and see them from an entirely new vantage point.

Our bodies have constantly changing moods, just like our minds, and these poses allow you to key into what's going on in it today. What is your body feeling? Are you stiff and sore, full of knots? Or are you pretty relaxed? Where is your mind? Are you present on the mat or are the lights on with nobody home? Are you stuck in your head? Maybe you feel energized, or maybe yoga is the last thing you feel like doing and you want to just run out of the room. But you've taken the first step and gotten yourself onto the mat, and that was the hardest thing you'll have to do. Now simply let go. The degree to which

you let go is the degree to which you allow the flow to begin.

If you are struggling, then on some level you are holding on. To what? Your anxieties. Your worries. Your tensions. Let go! If not now, when? Dissolve the walls, let go of your rope, and flow.

Remember, the answer to *how* is always *be in the now*. Follow your breath as it guides you into the present moment, and everything else will melt away like ice cubes in hot water. Just breathe and come into the present moment—the open doorway to that transformative space where all growing and healing happens.

Pose 1: *Child's Pose (Balasana)*

We open our practice by taking Child's Pose. As part of Integration, Child's Pose awakens the connection between your breath and your body and releases and relaxes all the muscles. But Child's Pose can also be home base for the duration of your practice. It is a resting pose that slows down the heart rate and provides full-body rest, allowing for deep restoration. Come to Child's Pose as often as you need during your practice. Beginning students may have to come here ten, twenty, a hundred times during their practice, and that's perfectly OK. Give yourself permission to do that, to take care of yourself. If you need to rest, just be true to yourself. No worries, no hurry—you'll get stronger in increments and build more stamina over time.

While Child's Pose is a resting pose, it

tively so that you are not in pain. You should be dynamically engaged but not strained.

Drop your head, drop your brain, and breathe—just being and breathing deep and free. Your ujjayi breath should be rhythmic, with an oceanic power. Let the layers of tension fall away one by one. Starting in this moment, let go!

Alignment:

- Contract and activate your quadriceps.
- Press your thighbones back toward the wall behind you.
- Pull your hips back and tilt your tailbone up.
- Lift your sitting bones upward toward the sky and spread them away from each other.
- Pull your navel toward your spine for upward lift.
- Press your arms down and forward.
- Drop the shoulder blades down your back, bringing elbows in toward each other.
- Palms should be flat, like pancakes, pressing your mat forward.
- Spread your fingers evenly apart.
- Place weight into your knuckles, not your wrists. Give emphasis to pressing down through the knuckles of your index fingers.

Risk Factor: Thrusting all your torso weight downward can jam your wrists and shoulders. Lift your chest and torso a few inches upward toward the ceiling to avoid this. Also, your wrists can strain if you are pushing them into the floor rather than pressing evenly into your hands and knuckles.

Modification: To relieve pressure on your wrists, triple-fold your mat and set it under the base of your palms. This will shift the weight into the knuckles and fingers and out of your wrists. Continue to rotate outward from your shoulder joints and press through the space between the thumb and index finger. Some beginners experience wrist pain until the muscles in their forearms, shoulders, and back are stronger, so have patience with yourself. You will get stronger very quickly if you practice daily.

Spiritual Focus: Small children aren't posing or posturing. They are just being. You can always tell when someone is posturing in a yoga pose. Just let yourself be natural. Naturalness starts with a willingness to come out from behind the mask: posturing less, letting go more, and just letting the light shine through us. This light is an invisible force that reaps visible results, ultimately allowing us to shine.

Pose 3: Ragdoll (Uttanasana)

Ragdoll, the final pose in the Integration series, continues to deeply release the back of your body as it awakens your biochemistry. Like Downward Facing Dog, it has an inversion element to it, which flushes your brain with fresh oxygen-rich blood and soothes and revitalizes the nervous system.

Building Blocks: From Downward Facing Dog, walk your feet up to your hands.

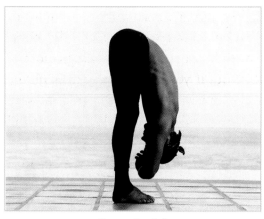
Pose 3: Ragdoll

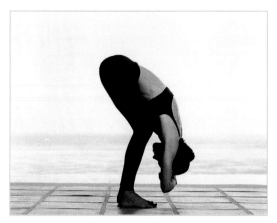
Ragdoll, modification

Your feet should be hip-width apart and parallel. Hinging at the hips, relax forward over your legs. Bring opposite hand to opposite bicep. Let your weight roll into the balls of your feet. Drop your head and let go of your neck. Spread your sitting bones away from each other as you hang forward. Your legs are strong, your upper body long, creating traction through your torso. Soften your eyes and set them on one point behind you.

Gently fan your toes and press the soles of your feet into your mat, creating that perfect rapport with the floor. Soften from the foundation of your feet upward. Walk the fingers of your mind up your calves, your knees, your hamstrings, your hips, all the way up your spine, adjusting your pose as needed along the way. If your lower back is stiff and asleep, breathe life into it. Nurture the opening of your entire body. Let your mask melt. Soften the contents of your skull.

Relax your neck and let the nectar flow to your brain. Shake your head "yes" and "no" a few times to make sure you're really relaxing. As you release the muscles in your neck, the artery that carries oxygen-rich blood to your brain dilates and the oxygen can flow freely to your brain. Your brain *loves* oxygen! It's so healthy to just hang upside down once in a while and give your brain a bath. Inverting your world clears the way for new viewpoints and insights. Wash away the old stuff, the limiting thoughts, the limiting beliefs, and come into your body with more compassion, more acceptance, more love and light. Be an open vessel and let the healing flow begin.

Hang down and just *breathe!*

Alignment:

- Keep your legs active and strong; the upper body is relaxed and free. Engage the quadriceps and lift the hamstrings upward.
- Let your head dangle, creating length through your neck.
- Bring your hips over your heels.

- Keep a slight bend in your knees to protect them and your lower back.
- Press your thighbones back and your sitting bones outward.

Risk Factor: If you feel strain in your lower back, take the modification below. If your legs are straight, be careful not to hyperextend the knees; keep them soft.

Modification: Bend your knees as much as you need to. There is no prize for straight legs!

Spiritual Focus: Sometimes by relaxing and doing nothing, great things can happen. At a certain point in his life, Gandhi didn't speak, he didn't really eat, he hardly wore any clothes. He refined his life to great simplicity, and through his powerful intention he changed the world.

2. Sun Salutations: Awakening

Sun Salutations are the full-body warm-ups that build heat and set the pace, breathing rhythms, and flow of your yoga practice. They bring your focus further inward and ignite the healing heat inside.

There are two Sun Salutation series: Sun Salutation A and Sun Salutation B, both of which are done with momentum in flowing sequence. They mobilize the musculature of the body, get the heart pumping, boost circulation, and prepare the body for the entire practice by taking each joint through its full range of motion.

Very often the first fifteen minutes of Sun Salutations will be filled with resistance. They may feel hard and uncomfortable. But if you keep moving through the poses and breathing in a conscious way, something will suddenly shift and you will enter a flow, a zone. At certain times you just don't feel "into it," but if you do it anyway, the energy shifts. You move to a new place and space, and suddenly you forget all the reasons why it was so hard at first and just start flowing. You come out of your head, dissolve resistance, and turn the faucet on. If you get an attack of doubt, just remember: You don't have to like it right in this moment, you just need to do it. Yoga practice is not always easy, but it is always necessary!

The Sun Salutations build purifying fire, but they also serve another important purpose. These two series play a key role in the flow of your entire practice. To maintain the flow, we often need connectors, or joining poses, that will lead us from one pose into the next. And that's where the Sun Salutations come in. They clean the slate between postures so you can start the next one neutralized and fresh. You'll come back to the Sun Salutation series again and again to keep the internal fire burning and to keep your practice flowing.

I'll break the poses down one by one, and then you can do the sequences as a flow.

Sun Salutation A
Pose 4: Samasthiti

There are several poses that we refer to only by their Sanskrit names, Samasthiti being one of them. This pose, which literally means "standing at attention," cultivates body awareness and develops new patterns of posture and personal stature. The alignment of Samasthiti is important because it is the blueprint for so many other poses; the rest are really just torso, arm, and leg variations of this central stature. Samasthiti is like the first note of a symphony—it all builds from there. The more conscious attention you give to this pose, the sweeter the music you will make.

Building Blocks: From Ragdoll, toe/heel your feet all the way together. With soft knees, slowly roll up to standing, one vertebra at a time. As you come up, sweep your arms up sideways and take a deep inhalation. Exhale and bring your hands to your heart center, in the middle of your chest, pressing your palms together. Release your hands and let them hang by your side.

Stand up straight with the inside edges of your feet touching. In this and in all poses, start with your attention at your feet. Work from a strong base and move upward. Keep rooting your feet firmly into the floor. Your feet should be wide awake, as if you were standing in a pan of espresso. Drive your legs down into the earth and lift your sternum to the sky, creating traction between the souls of your feet and the top of

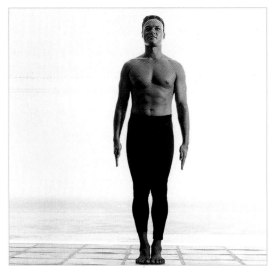

Pose 4: Samasthiti

your head. Root down, and your upper body automatically rebounds up. Bring some sunshine into your spine!

Gently contract your abdominal lock (uddiyana). Tip your tailbone down and under very slightly, centering your pelvis as though you are holding a bowl of water on the pelvic floor and do not want a single drop to spill over the front edge. Spin your inner thighs toward the wall behind you.

Pull the tops of your shoulders back and relax them. Your arms are alive and energized, palms facing inward. Beam energy down to the core of the earth through your fingertips. Keep your head centered and your neck neutral. Work the breath, stretching the exhalation. Be sound in wind and limb.

Stand tall with a natural integrity. Align your mind to your spine and just stand in that beautiful center line of gravity. Open your heart center. This pose begins with the inner posture of your mind, so lift your mind and your spine will follow. Consciously increase your personal stature. Let your body mold itself around your calm inner power.

- Root the soles of your feet to the earth and lift your arches.
- Spread all ten toes across the floor.
- Press the inner edges of your feet together.
- Engage your quads and press the leg bones down.
- Center your hips and scoop the front of your pelvis up as though you are holding water in the pelvic bowl.
- Open your chest and lift your sternum.
- Straighten and elongate your spine.
- Pull the tops of your shoulders back and relax them down, away from your ears.
- Energize your arms and face your palms inward.
- Activate your fingertips.
- Set your tranquil and soft gaze at a point straight ahead.

Risk Factor: Pushing your chest out like a drill sergeant puts strain on your spine and crunches the kidneys. Focus on keeping your ribs, spine, and hips in a natural and neutral alignment. Avoid hyperextending your knees.

Spiritual Focus: Your light shines most brightly when you drop your guard and dissolve the walls. The walls we put up to keep others out also keep us hidden within. Life is so short, why hide? Take up lots of space, relax your body, be open, and just doubt your doubts!

Pose 5: Mountain Pose (Tadasana)

Mountain pose reverses and relieves the constant gravitational stress on the body. It lengthens and creates openness in the front of the torso, neck, chest, and shoulders. We tend to compact our bodies as we go through the daily motions of life—sitting at the computer, carrying heavy packages and even kids, worrying and stressing our shoulders right up into our ears. There have been studies done that prove we are actually an average of one inch shorter at the end of each day due

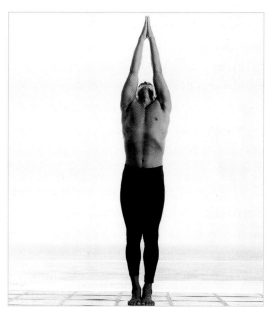

Pose 5: Mountain Pose

to compression in the spine. Cartilage reabsorbs water when we lie down at night and counteracts the day's shrinkage, but over time, the compression adds up. In life we compress, but in yoga we expand and release. This is why I focus so much on the elongation of the spine, pulling the torso up out of the pelvis, reaching toward the sky rather than giving in to gravity.

Your entire nervous system gets a wake-up call in this pose. All our nerves are in some way linked either directly or indirectly to the spinal column. It's the six degrees of separation as played out in the human body. As the spine naturally extends, the nerves are released from any pinching or compression and you can feel them lighting up like a Christmas tree.

Building Blocks: From Samasthiti, spin your palms outward. Inhale, lift your chin slightly, and sweep your hands up sideways, stopping when they are shoulder-width apart above your head. Your palms should be facing each other or pressed together. Gaze at a point directly above you on the ceiling. Tuck your tailbone under slightly and drop your front ribs downward. Be careful not to blow your rib cage out and up. Keep your arms straight and your palms facing each other.

Root into the ground through the soles of your feet and reach up to the sky through your fingertips. Engage the same traction as in Samasthiti. Be of heaven and earth, as grounded and soaring as a mountain!

Alignment:

Same as for Samasthiti, plus:

Reach your fingertips to the sky and root your feet down into the earth, creating length and space in your entire body.

Risk Factor: Watch out for an excessive arch in your back. Keep your spine neutral. When lifting your chin, do not strain your neck.

Spiritual Focus: You don't need people's permission or approval to act on what you know in your heart is right. Being in a state of grace means simply knowing what is right in the present moment and acting on it.

Pose 6: Standing Forward Bend (Uttanasana)

The forward-bending motion of Uttanasana stretches the lower back and hamstrings. Internally, it stimulates and rinses the organs in the belly, including the digestive system, and it ignites the metabolic fire. As with all forward bends, it harmonizes the brain chemistry.

Building Blocks: From Mountain pose, exhale and swan dive forward with a straight spine, hinging at your hips. Your arms sweep down sideways, stopping when your fingers reach the floor on either side of your feet. Press your chest down into your legs; Crazy Glue your nipples to your thighs. Ideally, your palms should be flat on the floor alongside the outsides of your

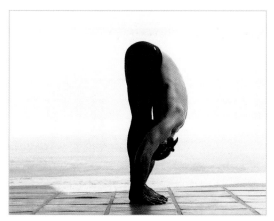
Pose 6: Standing Forward Bend

- Keep your feet active.
- Stack your shins, knees, thighbones, and hips in a vertical line.
- Sway your hips forward to line them up over your heels.
- Spread your sitting bones away from each other.
- Lengthen the front of the torso and spine downward.

Risk Factor: You can strain the lower back or hamstrings if you are tight in that area and bend too far.

Modification: As you bend forward, you can experiment with softening your knees to stabilize your lower back. Give emphasis to hinging at your hips and your abdominal lock. Once in the pose, bend your knees as much as you need to. If you are stiff, work with your feet slightly apart but still parallel.

Spiritual Focus: Resenting our present condition can cause us to try to "grab the bull by the horns" and struggle to get to success quickly. But just being in the present moment and playing your own edge is enough and allows you to grow naturally. It's like the story of the tortoise and the hare: The tortoise took slow and steady steps, and he achieved his goal before the pushy and fast-footed hare.

feet, but touching your fingertips to your mat is also fine (if you need to bend your knees, do so). Your head hangs down, your neck free, eyes soft.

Really focus on drawing the crown of your head down toward the mat, using your hands around your ankles as extra leverage if you want. Stretch the back of your legs to the sky and pull your trunk downward to the earth. Squeeze your legs and extend your spine. You should feel a good healthy stretch in your hamstrings and lower back. Increase the intensity smoothly, sensitively, and with total awareness.

If you are tight in your lower spine and hamstrings, this stretch may be intense at first, so bend your knees and focus on hinging at your hips. Just concentrate on breathing directly into any tightness and resistance you feel, allowing those areas to open up and release the tension stored there. This is a great diagnostic pose to determine the mood of your lower back on any given day.

The Halfway Lift continues to stretch the hamstrings and lower back, and it also elongates the spine and tones the abdominal obliques (the muscles that wrap around the sides of the abdominal wall).

Building Blocks: From Standing Forward Bend, keep your feet together and place your fingertips on the floor to the outer edges of your feet, in line with your toes. Inhale as you lift your torso halfway up to a flat back.

Each time you come into this position, you want to smooth out the lumps and bumps and iron out your spine. To do that, you need to work forward *and* backward, pressing your butt back and pulling your chest plate forward, creating traction from the crown of your head to your tailbone. The goal here is to create a beautiful lifeline through your spine, so bend your knees as much as you need in order to make this happen. Don't forget uddiyana: Pull your belly in and up.

Drop your shoulder blades down your back, away from your ears, and keep your chin tucked down. Focus your gaze at a spot on the floor six inches in front of your toes.

Alignment:

- Place your fingertips on the floor shoulder-width apart, in line with your toes.
- Press your pubic bone back and your chest forward.
- Extend and lengthen the spine; create traction from your tailbone to the crown of your head.
- Drop your shoulder blades down your back and away from your ears.
- Bring your chin down toward your chest so your neck is in one line with your entire spine.
- Gaze at the floor six inches ahead of your toes.

Risk Factor: Beware of jamming your chin up and crunching your neck. Your neck is a fragile creature, so keep it neutral and

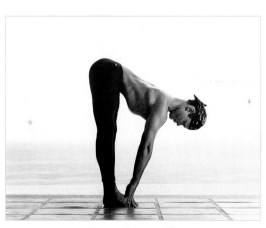

Pose 7: Halfway Lift

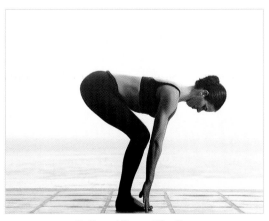

Halfway Lift, modification

treat it with love. Focus on pulling your shoulders away from your ears. Also, be sure to engage your abdominal lock (uddiyana) to protect your lower back.

Modification: Bend your knees if you are stiff, are rounding through your spine, or if this hurts your lower back.

Spiritual Focus: As a plant thrives in the warmth of the sun, so are you meant to be a creature of your intuitive light. Through that inner illumination, the power of the universe wordlessly suggests the way to go and grow. But through self-doubt your soul is cut off from that source and darkness whispers the way. Let your breath guide you back to your intuitive light, moment by moment.

Pose 8: Plank/High Push-Up (Dandasana)

High Push-Up builds upper and lower body integration. It strongly engages your biceps, triceps, shoulder, and chest muscles, as well as your abdominal obliques.

Building Blocks: From the Halfway Lift, bend your knees and, as you exhale, jump or walk your legs back to the top of a push-up position. Now set up your base. First things first: your eyes. Set the eyes at a spot between your hands. Bring your hands directly under your shoulders, stacking your shoulders, elbows, and wrists in one vertical line. Tuck your toes under and come onto the balls of your feet. Engage your quads and lift the front of your thighs, si-

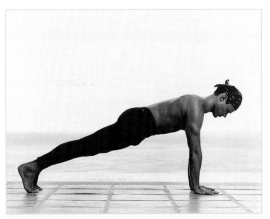

Pose 8: Plank/High Push-Up

multaneously pressing back through your heels. Lift your belly to your spine. Use your core power and your legs to help you hold this pose. Be strong. Be *powerful!*

There are two essential rotations happening at once in this pose: Your shoulder blades are spiraling down your back, away from your ears, and your tailbone is scooping down toward your heels, tilting your pelvis under slightly. These rotations will help stabilize your body instead of its collapsing against the force of gravity.

This can be a challenging pose, especially if you don't have a lot of upper body strength yet. But what you want to do is integrate as much of your musculature into this movement as possible, especially your quadriceps and abdominal muscles. If all the muscles in your body worked together, they would collectively have twenty-five tons of pulling power. Think of it! If your muscle power could conceivably pull ten gigantic trucks, it can certainly support however many pounds of you there are.

Even if it's hard, what is more challenging than this pose is what's going on inside your head. Are you calm, or are you resisting? Are you relaxed, or are you clenched? To stay calm in the face of adversity—to breathe more and struggle less, to be nonreactive—that's what is most challenging. It is also what is most essential to your success in the pose.

Alignment:

- Feet are hip-width apart.
- Curl your toes under so you are on the balls of your feet.
- Engage your quadriceps: enthusiasm through your thighs!
- Lift the front of your pelvis slightly up toward your chest.
- Gently lift and contract your abdomen.
- Stack your shoulder joints, elbows, and wrists all in one line.
- Slide your shoulders down your back.
- Gaze down to a spot between your hands.

Risk Factor: Don't let your shoulder blades collapse in toward each other and/or sink the lower back/belly down toward the floor. Keep your arms straight and your body lifted.

Modification: If you don't have enough upper body strength to hold this pose, drop your knees to the floor, but keep everything else the same. In time you will get stronger and be able to support your full body weight.

Spiritual Focus: When personal growth becomes the most important thing in our lives, we become committed to giving up our excuses and limiting thoughts like "I can't" and begin to find a way. Each moment of our practice is an opportunity to consciously rewire our belief system from doubt to faith, from confusion to knowing what is needed, both on and off the mat.

Pose 9: Low Push-Up (Chaturanga Dandasana)

Next in the Sun Salutation vinyasa is Chaturanga, or what I call "low push-up" position. Chaturanga Dandasana translates to "four-limbed staff," which is exactly what you want to look like in this pose: strong and straight. It should appear effortless, yet packed with power. Chaturanga encourages full-body stabilization and coordinated force.

Building Blocks: From High Push-Up, exhale and bend your elbows. Move forward as you lower your torso until you are hovering about five inches from the floor. Your elbows should form perfect 90-degree angles. Keep your elbows tucked into your sides and stacked directly over your wrists. Again, engage your belly and quads so you distribute the burden of weight more evenly. As in High Push-Up, tuck your tailbone down toward your heels. Keep your chin slightly raised.

A lot of students try to sneak their way past Low Push-Up and move directly from High Push-Up to the next pose,

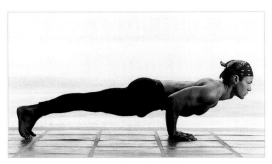

Pose 9: Low Push-Up

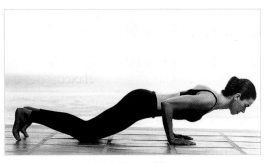

Low Push-Up, modification

which is Upward Facing Dog, but I strongly encourage you not to do this. Find ways to work within the pose. Modify, dilute, research, but don't run or avoid the work. Challenge yourself sensitively and your weakness will soon turn to strength. Each time you try it you will be able to go a little farther, or hover a little bit longer, but remember not to despise the days of small beginnings!

Alignment:
- Balance on the balls of the feet.
- Engage and lift your quads.
- Pull your belly up.
- Drop your shoulder blades down the back. Keep your shoulders square, not rounded forward.
- Stack your elbows over your wrists and tuck them into your ribs.
- Shoulders hover at elbow level.
- Gently lift your chin.
- Set a powerful gaze forward.

Risk Factor: You can strain your shoulders by letting your elbows fall out to the sides. Keep your arms tucked in close to your body. You can also put excessive strain on your elbow joints by dipping your shoulders lower than elbow height. Many people crunch the neck and upper back (as well as strain their wrists) by allowing their mid-torso to sag. Keep as straight as a staff!

Modification: As in High Push-Up, drop your knees until you build more upper body strength. If you need further modification, drop your chest down to the floor.

Spiritual Focus: The staff is symbolic of great power, strength, and leadership. When Moses led the Jews out of Egypt, the Pharoah's army had trapped them at the Red Sea. But Moses raised his staff and parted the Red Sea so his people could walk through and escape. When you find yourself stuck or stagnant, raise the staff of your spirit and watch as that which blocked your path *becomes* the path.

Pose 10: Upward Facing Dog
(Urdhva Mukha Svanasana)
Upward Facing Dog stretches the entire front of your torso and continues to

strengthen the muscles in your arms, shoulders, and back. It also opens the chest, which expands your ability to breathe more deeply twenty-four hours a day.

Building Blocks: From Low Push-Up, inhale and press down on your hands, scooping your chest and belly up. Your hands should be flat, like pancakes. Move your torso forward and through your arms, which will cause you to roll over the tops of your toes so your feet are pointed with the tops pressing into your mat. Point all ten toes backward as if each one had a tiny pin of light on the tip and you wanted to shine ten spotlights on the wall behind you. Pull your shoulders back, your chest high. Enthusiasm through your thighs! Press down through the palms of your hands and the tops of your feet. Squeeze your butt and legs so your upper thighs are lifted off the mat. Your inner thighs spin upward and your baby toes touch the floor.

Drop your shoulders down your back, away from your ears. The shoulder blades are like hands pushing your chest forward from behind. Lift and open your chest plate—breathe deep and free into the bottom of your lungs. Pull your heart muscle away from your heels. Create length and space in your spine; drive down through your arms and feet, really arching up. Pull your mat back with your hands as you lift your chest higher. It should feel so good to stretch out and expand the whole front side of your hips and upper body.

Gaze forward and shine!

Alignment:

- Press your palms and the tops of your feet down into your mat.
- Engage your quadriceps, glutes, and abdomen to lift the front of your thighs off your mat.
- Spin your inner thighs up, keeping your toes on the floor.
- Stack your shoulders, elbows, and wrists in one vertical line.
- Shoulders should be square, not rounded forward.
- Chest and torso should be slightly in front of your hands.

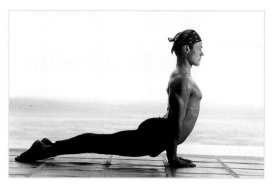

Pose 10: Upward Facing Dog

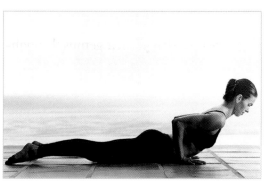

Upward Facing Dog, modification

- Let your torso hang like a pendulum between your arms.
- Your head, shoulders, and chest should be in a neutral position, just as if you were standing upright.
- Increase the space between your shoulders and ears.
- Keep your neck neutral, in line with the spine.
- Set a soft and steady gaze forward.

Risk Factor: Beware of collapsing into your low back. Maintain the stabilization and action of your arms, legs, glutes, and belly to prevent this.

Modification: Bend your elbows, tuck them into your sides, and let your navel and thighs come down to the mat until you build more upper body strength and suppleness.

Spiritual Focus: Goal-driven creation stifles our true brilliance and ability. The gift of great geniuses is their ability to access and express the deep creative potential that speaks to all of us. As we access this inner energy daily, we can express it outwardly in the same way that da Vinci, Mozart, or Shakespeare radiated their genius throughout the world.

Repeat Pose 2: Downward Facing Dog (Adho Mukha Svanasana)

You already know how to set up the alignment within Downward Facing Dog from the Integration Series. However, Downward Facing Dog is also an integral part of the Sun Salutations vinyasa. To move into Downward Facing Dog from Upward Facing Dog, exhale, and in one fluid motion let the power of your thighs pull you back into your inverted "V." Adjust your hands and feet as necessary.

In Sun Salutations, hold Downward Facing Dog for five full breaths.

Pose 11: Jump Forward

The Jump Forward is a link between one pose and another. Remember, the poses between poses are poses! This creates a mobile flexibility and strength and helps to keep building heat.

Building Blocks: On the fifth exhalation in Downward Facing Dog, empty your lungs completely and press your thighs back even farther. Pull your belly up to your spine. Look at your hands, bend your knees, and, using your abdominal stability and upper body force, jump your feet forward between your hands. The objective is to be light and easy, not to plunk forward like an elephant. Don't use momentum; just float!

The Jump Forward is a combination of moving strength, fluid flexibility, equal balance, and arm and torso stabilization. The weightless quality of floating forward is something that comes through practice and progress. Just keep practicing, keep practicing, and then one day you'll just levitate forward effortlessly and say, "Wow, where did that come from?!"

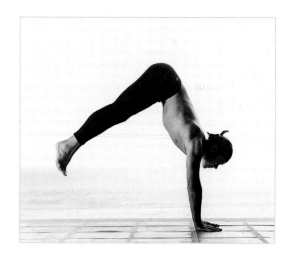

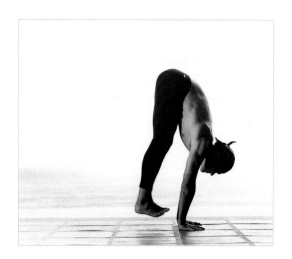

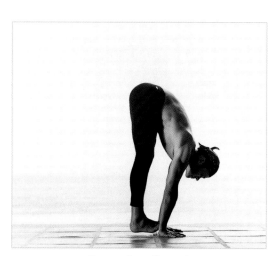

Pose 11: Jump Forward

Modification: Walk your feet forward one foot at a time until you are more comfortable with the jump.

Spiritual Focus: This movement helps you discover what I call your "midair mind." Remember what it was like to jump over a puddle when you were a kid? There was a split second between when you left one side and before you landed on the other when you were suspended in midair. Spiritually, that is the moment of pure freedom—of just *being*.

To Finish the Sun Salutation Vinyasa A:

Once you Jump Forward, come into Halfway Lift (pose 7), then fold down into Standing Forward Bend (6). From there, sweep your arms up sideways and then into Mountain Pose (5). Be sure to engage your abdominal lock as you sweep up to the sky. Then drop your arms and come back to Samasthiti (4).

Overview of Sun Salutation/Vinyasa A:

Samasthiti
Mountain Pose (inhale)
Standing Forward Bend (exhale)
Halfway Lift (inhale)
Jump (or walk) back (exhale)
High Push-Up (inhale)
Low Push-Up (exhale)
Upward Facing Dog (inhale)
Downward Facing Dog (press back on the
    exhale and inhale, exhale five times)
Jump Forward (hold exhale)
Halfway Lift (inhale)

From here forward, we will refer to the Sun Salutation A series as "Vinyasa A." Repeat the entire Vinyasa A series three to five times before moving on to the next series, Sun Salutation B.

Sun Salutation B

Now that you've started to warm up, we move to Sun Salutation B, which turns the internal heat up a little higher. Much of this vinyasa is the same as Sun Salutation A, with a few new poses included.

Pose 12: Thunderbolt (Utkatasana)

Utkatasana translates to "powerful" or "mighty"—just like a thunderbolt. The dynamic quality of this pose increases the heart rate and stimulates the circulatory and metabolic systems. It is a great toner for the back, butt, hips, and thighs, and also stretches the Achilles tendons and shins.

Building Blocks: From Samasthiti, inhale as you bend your knees down deep to 90 degrees and bring your hands up over your head, arms alongside your ears. Squat down as if you were sitting in a chair, bringing your hips/tail slightly back. Lift your toes off the floor and shift the majority of your body weight (80 percent) back to your heels. You want to create lower body strength, upper body length, and space. Hips low, heart high. Squeeze your sitting muscles in toward each other and lengthen your spine, reaching your arms up like a thunderbolt.

Spread your shoulder blades apart. Pull your fingers up out of their knuckles. Spin your pinky fingers in toward each other, rotating your thumbs outward. Gently lift your chin and look up through your hands.

It may feel a little stressful to hold this for the full five breaths, but as I've said, sometimes your stress reduction program is going to be a little bit stressful! In moments of stress in life, we tend to tense up and breathe less. But when in the middle of stress—in life or in this pose—you have the perfect opportunity to reverse that pattern and rewire your nervous system. Rather than breathing less in stress, breathe more.

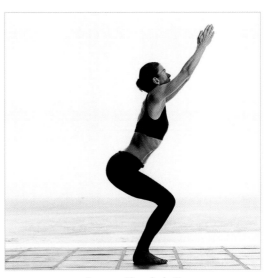

Pose 12: Thunderbolt

- Lift your toes and shift 80 percent of your weight onto your heels.
- Maintain strong legs.
- Keep your hips/tail slightly back.
- Drop your hips and lift your heart and hands.
- Pull your arms up through your fingertips.
- Spin your arms so your little fingers move in and your thumbs move outward.
- Spread your scapulae and broaden your upper back.
- Set your eyes at a point between your hands.

Risk Factor: Shifting your weight forward toward your toes stresses the knees.

Modification: The lower your hips, the more intense the pose, so bend or straighten your knees to whatever degree is comfortable for you.

Spiritual Focus: Calm determination is the difference between being stuck and being struck with a lighting power from within. Willing your way toward success in this pose or in anything in life will almost always create suffering. Stay with the moment-by-moment calm determination and you will signal the unseen and mysterious forces that you are serious about growth. Like a magnet you will attract them.

Connecting Vinyasa

After the fifth breath of Thunderbolt, lower your hips two more inches for one additional breath, then exhale and hinge forward. Go through steps six through ten of Vinyasa A (Standing Forward Bend, Halfway Lift, High Push-Up, Low Push-Up, Upward Facing Dog) and end in Downward Facing Dog (2).

Pose 13: Warrior I (Virabhadrasana I)

Warrior I creates a powerful integration of leg strength with fluid flexibility of the hips. It also prepares the body for backbends later in the practice.

Building Blocks: From Downward Facing Dog, exhale and lunge your right foot forward between your hands, bending your front knee to 90 degrees. Spin your back foot flat to a 60-degree angle, with your heels in one line. Take a moment to build your house on a rock. Check that your heels are in one line to create a stable foundation. On the in breath, sweep your hands up over your head, again on either side of your ears. Face your palms toward each other with the little fingers spinning in, the thumbs spinning out.

Continue to square your hips, pulling your right hip back and your left hip forward. Both thighbones rotate in a clockwise direction. Dip your hips down until your thigh is parallel to the floor— you should be able to balance an orange on the top of your front thigh. The back leg should be strong, like steel! Keep your right knee stacked over your right ankle; the right knee moves right, pressing toward your right baby toe. Press

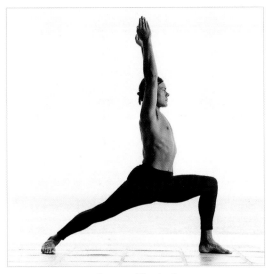

Pose 13: Warrior I

down through the outer edge of your back foot.

Pull your sternum upward, as though the point two inches below the soft spot between your collarbones was attached to a string suspended from the ceiling. Lift your heart without blowing your ribs up and out. Soften the front ribs downward and your whole spine will lengthen. Your shoulders are relaxed, they lift up, and your arms reach high. Take aim and set your eyes straight ahead.

Alignment:
- Heels in one line.
- Your back foot is flat and turned in to a 60-degree angle.
- Lift your inner ankle and press into the outer edge of your back foot.
- Dip your front leg down to 90 degrees so the thigh and shin form a right angle.
- Center and lift the front of your pelvis.

- Scoop your tailbone down and forward.
- Rotate both femur bones in a clockwise direction from the hip socket for the right side, counterclockwise for the left.
- Pull your belly in.
- Lift your heart to the heavens.
- Reach your arms up.
- Set your eyes straight ahead.

Risk Factor: Pushing your chest and ribs forward compresses the mid-spine and the kidneys.

Modification: If this pose is too intense, lessen the width of your stance and straighten your front knee to a comfortable degree.

Spiritual Focus: Your presence in this pose can be as empty or as soulful as you make it. You can get all caught up in the mechanics and stay in your head, or you can drop your brain, follow your breath into the "now moment," and rise above the battlefield of your mind. Be a warrior, not a worrier!

Connecting Vinyasa

From Warrior I, place your hands down on your mat and step back into High Push-Up (8) position. Go through Vinyasa A (High Push-Up, Low Push-Up, Upward Facing Dog, Downward Facing Dog). From Downward Facing Dog, step your left foot forward and spin your right foot flat into Warrior I, following all the same instructions as above, except in reverse.

Go through the Vinyasa A again (High to Low Push-Up, Upward Facing Dog to Downward Facing Dog). Take five deep breaths in Downward Facing Dog. On the last breath, exhale completely and Jump Forward (11). Inhale and Halfway Lift (7), then Forward Bend (6), bend your knees and sweep back up again into Thunderbolt (12). Hold Thunderbolt for five breaths, then fold forward into Standing Forward Bend (6) and begin another Sun Salutation B from there.

Repeat Sun Salutation B (Vinyasa B) two times. For the third round, add in the next pose, Warrior II.

Overview of Sun Salutation/Vinyasa B:

Thunderbolt (inhale)

Standing Forward Bend (exhale)

Halfway Lift (inhale), exhale as you step back

High Push-Up (inhale)

Low Push-Up (exhale)

Upward Facing Dog (inhale)

Downward Facing Dog (exhale)

Warrior I, right foot forward (inhale)

High Push-Up, Low Push-Up, Upward Facing Dog, Downward Facing Dog

Warrior I, left foot forward (inhale)

High Push-Up, Low Push-Up, Upward Facing Dog, Downward Facing Dog

Jump Forward

Thunderbolt (inhale)

Pose 14: Warrior II (Virabhadrasana II)

Warrior II is an amazing hip-opening pose. It isometrically sculpts the muscles in the buttocks and thighs. Beyond that,

though, it hones your power of concentration. Through your focused gaze, this pose teaches you how to streamline your power into a single ray of energy.

On the third round of Vinyasa B, we add in Warrior II. Follow the entire sequence until you reach Warrior I (right foot forward), then instead of coming down into High Push-Up, come into Warrior II as follows:

Building Blocks: From Warrior I, square your hips and chest to the side wall (the left wall if your right foot is forward, and vice versa) and float your arms down to shoulder height until your arms are parallel with the floor. Your front arm should be aligned directly above the front thigh, the back arm in line with the back leg. Create a tug-of-war between your arms, as if you were being pulled apart at your wrists.

Check your heels—they should still be

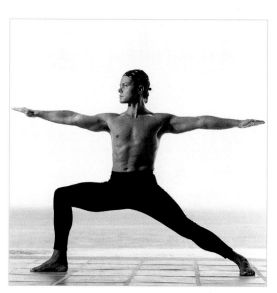

Pose 14: Warrior II

in one line. Give yourself a wide base. Dip your hips down, stacking the right knee over the ankle and moving it toward the right baby toe. As in Warrior I, the shin is vertical. Rotate your inner thighs away from each other. Create a center line by stacking your shoulders over your hips. Work maximum power through your arms and legs. Your front and back limbs should be opposing each other.

Drop your brain. Drop your shoulders. Lift and open your heart center. Focus your concentrated gaze on your front middle fingernail and breathe deep and free.

Alignment:

- Press through the outer edge of your back foot.
- Stretch the mat apart with your feet.
- Stack the front knee over the ankle.
- Dip your hips down so the front thigh is parallel to the floor.
- Squeeze your back leg and lift the back inner thigh to the sky.
- Spin your inner thighs out and away from each other.
- Press your tailbone toward your front knee.
- Lift your belly, spine, and chest.
- Stack your shoulders over your hips.
- Drop your shoulder blades down your back.
- Reach through both arms and fingertips, as if you were being pulled apart.
- Fuse your eyes to your front middle fingernail.

Risk Factor: Letting the front leg cave inward strains the knee. Keep your knee moving out toward the baby toe. Bending the back knee is also risky for the joint.

Modification: As in Warrior I, shorten your stance and straighten your knee to a comfortable degree.

Spiritual Focus: Beam your attention to a single focal point and you will feel your whole body glow with a life force. Concentrate and you will radiate!

Connecting Vinyasa

After five breaths in Warrior II, helicopter your back arm around to the floor and step back to High Push-Up (8) position. Go through Vinyasa B again (Low Push-Up, Upward Facing Dog, Downward Facing Dog) until you come into Warrior I with your left foot forward, and repeat Warrior II on the left side. Then follow the remaining steps of Vinyasa B (High Push-Up, Low Push-Up, Upward Facing Dog, Downward Facing Dog, Jump Forward, Thunderbolt). Finish by coming to Samasthiti.

3. Warrior Series: Vitality

Now that you're warmed up we start fanning the internal purifying flame. The Warrior series consists of seven very dynamic poses, all of which bring your heart rate up and get the energy flowing more vigorously.

For the first four poses in this series —Crescent Lunge, Revolving Crescent

Lunge, Extended Side Angle, and Side Plank—we do just the right side only, one time through as a flow. Then we go through a connecting vinyasa and flow through all four poses again, this time on the left side. The next three poses of this series—Prayer Twist, Gorilla, and Crow—are done individually with connecting steps in between.

Pose 15: Crescent Lunge (Anjaneyasana)

Crescent Lunge is a full-body pose that trains all the muscles to work as a team. It creates a flexible strength and tone through the lower body, stability in the front and back of the torso, and length through the upper body.

Building Blocks:

Part one: Go through Vinyasa A until you are in Downward Facing Dog. From here, bring your right leg up to the sky. Roll your hip open and reach your right foot high, as though you were going to bring it over and around to reach your left shoulder. Reach through your foot, fan your toes, drop your head, and hold for five breaths.

Part two: After the fifth exhalation, square your hips back to center, look up, and step your right foot forward between your hands and bend your right knee to 90 degrees (as though you were going into Warrior I). Lunge deep! Leave your back heel up so you are standing on the ball of the back foot. Both feet are now facing forward. You want your feet about four inches apart in width. If your feet are in one line, you'll be on a tightrope and it will be difficult to balance. Tuck your tail under. Inhale and sweep your arms up over your head with your palms facing each other, again as in Warrior I. Reach up

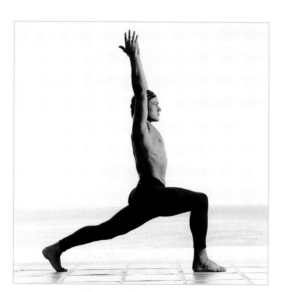

Pose 15: Crescent Lunge

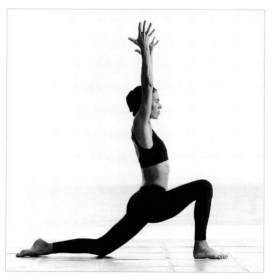

Crescent Lunge, modification

through your fingertips, pinkies turning in, thumbs turning out.

Set your foundation by pressing through the balls of both feet, stretching the mat apart between them. As in Warrior I, keep the front knee moving out toward the right baby toe. Lift the back quadricep and knee to the ceiling to straighten your back leg. Your back leg is the anchor here; keep it strong!

Gently lift and contract your abdomen to stabilize your core. There is a balance element to this pose, so get a sense of your center. Pull your right hip back, your left hip forward, squaring your hips so that they face the wall in front of you. Align your mind to your spine so you move and breathe from your center of balance.

The entire upper half of your body should mimic Mountain pose: Pull your shoulders down and away from your ears. Reach your spine, sternum, arms, and fingertips up. Find the traction of lower body strength and upper body length.

Full body expression here: All four limbs are alive and active. Your whole body should be animated with breath and energy!

Alignment:
- Maintain a four-inch width between your feet.
- Dip your hips until your front knee is at a 90-degree angle.
- Keep your front knee stacked over the ankle and moving out toward the baby toe.
- Back leg straight, quadricep and knee lifting toward the ceiling.

- Drive your tailbone forward and lift the front of your pelvis upward.
- Soften your front ribs down toward your belly.
- Bring your arms up in line with your ears.
- Reach up through your fingertips.
- Soften your eyes and fuse them to one point in front of you.

Risk Factor: Be mindful not to let the front knee fall in, which will put strain on it; keep it moving toward the baby toe. Don't thrust your ribs forward; this will crunch your mid-back.

Modification: Drop your back knee to your mat to reduce the intensity of this movement.

Spiritual Focus: Stress can be challenging, but stress can give life. A flower grows because of the sun, the wind, and the rain. The flower draws its life from these vital elements, but also draws its strengths from these same elements, which can beat cruelly upon it. It draws energy from the stress of the sun, wind, and rain. The flower grows not only *because of* these elements, but also *in spite of* them!

Pose 16: Revolving Crescent Lunge (Parivrtta Alanasana)

Twisting or spiraling the torso is one of the most powerful actions that you can do to transform the health of your internal organs, glands, circulatory system, muscles, and connective tissue. A deep twist squeezes and rinses out the organ or specific body part like a wet facecloth. After you finish a twisting action, the body part is flushed with fresh oxygen-rich blood, which washes away toxins and tensions.

This pose is like a tremendous massage. It rings out the lower back and the digestive and vital organs of the mid-body (liver, spleen, kidneys). Plus, this opens the chest and stretches the pectoral minor muscles, which are typically the tightest muscles in the body.

Building Blocks:

Part one: From Crescent Lunge, reach up a little farther through your hands, and as you exhale bring your hands together at your heart center in a prayerlike position (this is called Namaste). Exhale and spin your left arm to the outside of the right thigh. Keep your back heel lifted, your back leg straight and contracted, and the front knee stacked over the ankle. Leave some space between your torso and your front thigh. Press your palms together flat.

This is a twisting motion, and all twisting motions are done actively, meaning we extend the spine on the inhalation and twist open a little more on the exhalation. Press your lower arm against your outer thigh to leverage the twist. Pull your belly in as you spin. Pull the upper lung and shoulder blade back and press your lower shoulder forward. Be mindful of creating space in your middle and lower back here. Pull your shoulders down and away from your ears. Stretch your chest toward your

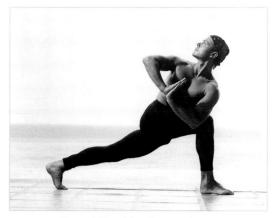
Pose 16: Revolving Crescent Lunge

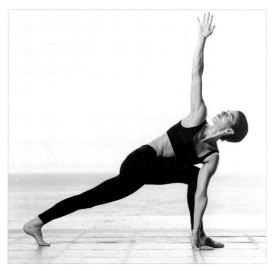
Revolving Crescent Lunge, arms extended

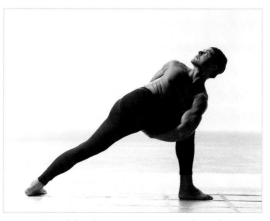
Revolving Crescent Lunge, arms bound

chin. Look up toward the ceiling (or down at the floor, if that feels better on your neck). Hold for five breaths.

Part two: Straighten your arms, bringing your lower hand to the floor on the outside of your front foot and your upper hand to the sky. Everything else stays the same. Upper shoulder blade pulls toward the spine, upper lung pulls back. Set your eyes on the upper thumbnail. Open the chest wide and breathe in all that life-giving oxygen! To make the pose more challenging, see if you can bind your arms by bringing your right hand behind your back and reaching through your legs with your left. Try to hook your hands or grab a wrist.

Alignment:

Same as for Crescent Lunge, plus:

- Pull your wrists back so they are aligned with your elbows to stabilize your upper body (part one).
- Press through both arms.
- Stack your upper hand directly over your shoulder and keep it active.
- Stretch every bone and muscle in your chest.
- Pull the hip of the front leg back and your chest toward your chin, creating traction through your torso.
- Drop your shoulder blades down your back.
- Gaze high, to the thumb of the upper hand.

Risk Factor: Same as for Crescent Lunge, plus wrenching your middle/lower back by twisting past a healthy point. Stay alert and aware of that part of your body and don't push too far past your edge.

Modification: As in Crescent Lunge, drop the back knee to make this movement easier. If you cannot bring your hand to the outside of your front foot, place it on the floor to the inside of the front foot, directly under your shoulder, or place your hand on a block.

Spiritual Focus: A baby chick develops the strength and vigor it needs to survive in the world by the very act of pecking, pushing, and twisting its way out of its protective shell. If you broke the shell open for the baby chick, it would not survive, because it did not go through its own process of struggle and freedom. Remember, the prize is in the process!

Pose 17: Extended Side Angle
(Utthita Parsvakonasana)

Extended Side Angle is another full-body pose that opens, stretches, and strengthens the whole body and integrates it as one unit. It cultivates balance and co-ordination. Specifically, it strengthens the muscles that stabilize the knees, sculpts the legs, and opens the chest.

Building Blocks: From Revolving Crescent Lunge, exhale as you place both hands on the floor to the inside of the front foot. Turn your back foot flat (as in Warrior I), heels in one line. Keep your right palm flat on your mat in line with your ankle and

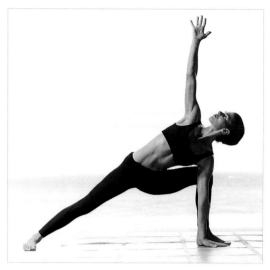

Pose 17: Extended Side Angle

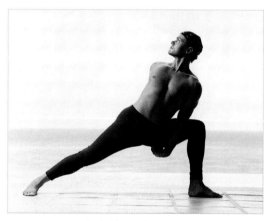

Extended Side Angle, arms bound

on the in breath reach and extend your spine, on the out breath rinse and spin. It's very important that you keep your tailbone tucked under and your chest lifting up. A common mistake many students will make is to thrust their butt backward and let their torso drop forward, which puts a lot of strain on the lower back and front knee. Try to keep your heels, hips, and head all on one plane. Your hips and your nipples are like headlights shining on the side wall. To make the pose more challenging, see if you can bind your arms by bringing your left hand behind your back and reaching through your legs with your right. Try to hook your hands or grab a wrist.

Alignment:

- Heels are in one line. Keep your feet full of life!
- Press the outer edge of your back foot into the mat.
- Draw the front hip in toward the center line.
- Scoop your tailbone down toward the back heel.
- Engage your back thigh, keeping the leg straight and strong.
- Stack your upper shoulder over the lower.
- Open your chest and give your lungs space to expand fully.
- Set your eyes up toward the sky.

Risk Factor: You can strain the lower back by allowing the butt to move back and the chest forward and down. Also, be mindful not to let the front knee fall inward.

exhale as you twist your torso and extend your left arm up to the sky. Use your lower elbow to nudge the knee to the right, and pull your right hip in and under so you can stack your torso on top of your right thigh. Press your lower shoulder forward and your upper shoulder back. Create traction from the palm of your lower hand to the extended fingertips of your raised arm. Set your gaze on your upper thumbnail.

This is another twisting movement, so

Modification: If it is difficult to keep your torso stacked over your thigh, set your front forearm on the top of your front thigh or place your lower hand on a block.

Spiritual Focus: You can reach and fight and strain your way through a pose if you so choose. Muscling through it might work for a while, but eventually it will catch up to you and tire you. At a certain point in your practice you get that there is an easier way—that exceeding yourself isn't about reaching or grasping but about melting into a new realm, a dimension of power that can do for us what we cannot do for ourselves.

Connecting Vinyasa

From the Extended Side Angle, bring your upper arm back down and place both palms on the floor, hands directly under your shoulders. Step back into High Push-Up (8). You are now set in position for the next pose, Side Plank.

Pose 18: Side Plank (Vasisthasana)

By using your own body weight as resistance in this pose, you tone and strengthen your arms and the front and back of your torso. Side Plank integrates the upper and lower body and further trains all the muscles in the body to work as one coordinated force.

Building Blocks: From High Push-Up, bring your feet all the way together so your inner thighs are touching. Spin your heels to the right and bring your left hand up to the sky. Your lower hand should be directly under your shoulder. Keep your upper hand active.

Proper alignment is essential to keeping your balance in this pose. You want to imagine your body is pressed between two panes of glass, one against the front and one against the back. Stack your upper hip directly over the lower one, and keep your heels, hips, and heart all in one line. Align your upper arm above your lower, stacking all the joints along one plane.

Don't just thrust all your weight onto your one little wrist; enlist all the muscles in your body. Flex your feet, contract your legs, and activate your abdominal lock (uddiyana) to stabilize the pose. There are two lines of traction happening at the same time: from the crown of your head to the soles of your feet, and from the palm pressing into your mat through your raised fingertips. Pull the front of your pelvis up

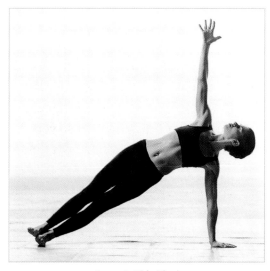

Pose 18: Side Plank

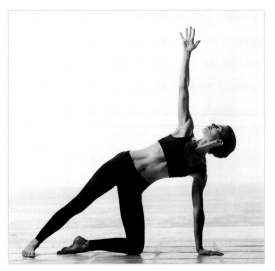

Side Plank, modification

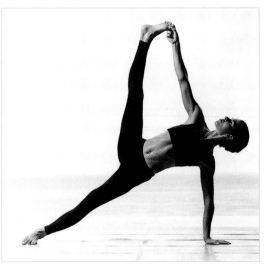

Side Plank, modification

toward your chest, and pull your heart muscle up toward your chin. Move your shoulders away from your ears to create more length and space. Reach your upper arm high to create lift and traction away from the bottom hand.

Turn your gaze to the thumbnail of your upper hand (or to your lower thumbnail if that feels better on your neck). Breathe deep and free through your whole body.

Alignment:

- Imagine your body being pressed between two panes of glass.
- Stack your heels, hips, and heart all in one line.
- Loop your tailbone toward your heels.
- Stack your upper hip directly above the lower.
- Lift your hips high; don't let them collapse down.

- Line up all the joints in your arms along one plane.
- Press your arms away from each other to create extension and traction through your chest, shoulders, and arms.
- Drop your shoulder blades down your back, away from your ears.
- Open your chest.
- Gaze high, to the upper thumbnail.

Risk Factor: Letting your upper body and pelvis sink down puts undo pressure on your wrist, shoulder, and neck. Don't press your chest too far forward in an attempt to open it; this will create an arch in your back and prevent your body from staying on one plane.

Modification: If this is difficult, drop your lower knee to the floor directly underneath the hip and spin your upper foot flat on the floor. If your knee is dropped, your right hand, knee, and back foot should all be in one line.

Spiritual Focus: Yoga practice is an unlearning process. We have to unlearn all that we've believed and been told about ourselves. Start believing what you know in your heart to be right; start trusting the teacher within. Start trusting what you see, know, and feel.

Connecting Vinyasa

Roll open a little more and then gently come back down to High Push-Up (8) and go through the movements of Vinyasa A until you come into Downward Facing Dog. Hold Downward Facing Dog for five breaths, then extend your left leg to the sky. Roll the hip open and bend the upper knee, reaching the left foot toward the right shoulder for five breaths. Then square your hips and lunge your left foot forward and go through the left-side sequence of Crescent Lunge (15), Revolving Crescent Lunge (16), Extended Side Angle (17), and Side Plank (18). After the second Side Plank, come back to High Push-Up and go through Vinyasa A once again, ending in Standing Forward Bend (6). From here bend your knees, dip your hips down, and lift your arms up to Thunderbolt (12). This sets you up for the next pose, which is the Prayer Twist.

Pose 19: Prayer Twist (Parivrtta Utkatasana)

This pose creates flexible strength in the mid- and lower back. It squeezes and rinses the organs and muscles of the mid-section of the body like a sponge, including the kidneys and digestive organs. Like all twisting poses, Prayer Twist is a powerful way to detoxify organs and glands, which boosts your overall health. Isometrically, it sculpts your buttocks, thighs, and back muscles.

Building Blocks: From Thunderbolt, reach up through your hands, and as you exhale bring them down into a prayerlike position at your heart. Inhale and spin your left elbow to the outside of your right thigh. Keep your feet and knees together and dip your hips low. Pull your butt back and your chest plate forward, lengthening your spine. Pull your sitting bones in toward each other.

Now straighten your arms. Ideally the lower hand comes to the floor with your five fingertips set into the floor, like a claw. You can use a block if you need to or, if you are more flexible, set your palm flat on the floor. Bring your right hand straight up to the sky, stacking it directly above your right shoulder. Bring your lower shoulder blade forward and pull your upper shoulder blade back. Look up and start to work your twist.

Match your breath to each micromovement. On the inhalation, lengthen the spine; on the exhalation, twist your torso open. Revolve on the out breath and rinse and massage your internal organs. On the in breath relax and feel the organs being flushed and bathed with fresh blood. Every two or three breaths, see if you can spin

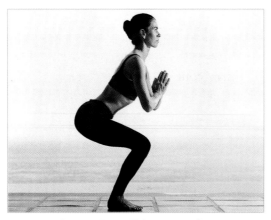
Pose 19: Prayer Twist, preparation

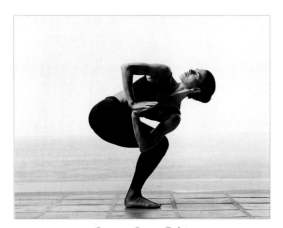
Pose 19: Prayer Twist

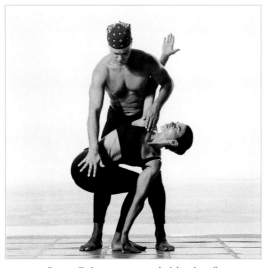
Prayer Twist, arms extended (assisted)

just a little bit more. Be sure to twist from your torso, not from your arms.

Alignment:
- Feet are together.
- Maintain strong legs.
- Keep your knees level and together.
- Dip your hips low.
- Squeeze your sitting bones and inner thighs in toward each other.
- Press your hips/tail back and pull your chest forward.
- Twist from your torso, not from your arms.
- Stack your upper shoulder over the lower shoulder.
- Create traction from fingertip to fingertip if your arms are extended, or elbow to elbow if your hands are at Namaste.
- Gaze high to the heavens.

Modification: Set your lower hand on a block. Also, look down if gazing high strains your neck.

Spiritual Focus: Putting actions to your intentions is the same as putting postures to your prayers. Let your intention for growth flow through your movements. Relax and ask for guidance and support and you will receive it.

Connecting Vinyasa

Hold this pose for a full five breaths, then relax into Ragdoll (3). Toe/heel your feet till hip-width apart and just hang forward for a few breaths. Then toe/heel your feet back together, sweep up to Thunderbolt (12) once again and do the same steps for Prayer Twist, except in reverse (bringing your right arm to the outside of your left thigh). After five breaths, again relax to Ragdoll, which puts you in position for the next pose, which is Gorilla.

Pose 20: Gorilla Pose (Padahastasana)

This deep forward bend releases the lower back and the backs of the legs. It is a potent counterpose that restores balance to your biochemistry, unclutters your mind, and allows you to slip into a calm state of concentration.

Building Blocks: From Ragdoll, place your hands all the way under your feet, palms up. Walk your toes up to your wrists, bending your knees as needed. Inhale and lift halfway up, working your way toward a flat back, then exhale and fold down, hinging from your hips. Straighten the knees inch by inch into a deep stretch.

Now, move your hips slightly forward, bringing your hips over your heels.

Breathe into your hamstrings. Play your edge—explore how far forward you can shift your weight to increase the intensity.

Relax your head and let gravity do its work. Just let go and breathe.

Alignment:
- Keep your feet hip-width apart and parallel.
- Walk your toes up so they are touching the insides of your wrists.
- Drop your head.
- Soften your face.
- Keep your eyes open and set on a point directly behind you.

Modification: Bend your knees as much as you need to.

Spiritual Focus: There once was a great magician who lived at the top of a cliff. One day, a couple who had been searching far and wide for peace and happiness climbed to where the magician lived, hoping he could provide them with what they were seek-

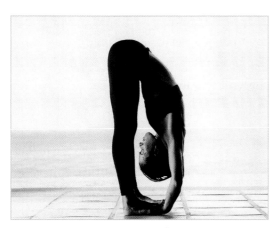

Pose 20: Gorilla

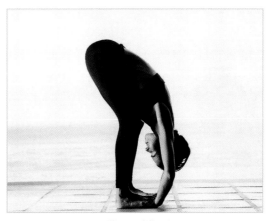

Gorilla, modification

ing. When they reached the top, they saw him standing on the edge of the cliff looking over and called to him.

"You must come to the edge," he said.

"No," they replied. "We are afraid. We will pay you to come to us and tell us what you know."

"You must come to the edge," the magician repeated. "It is the only way."

Trembling with fear, they stepped up to the edge. The magician put his hands on their shoulders. They believed he was trying to comfort them, but instead he pushed them off the edge . . . and they flew!

"All you needed was already within you," the magician said with a knowing smile.

Connecting Vinyasa

After five breaths, inhale and lift halfway up. As you exhale, release your hands and place them flat on the floor for the next pose, Crow.

Pose 21: Crow (Bakasana)

Crow is the pose I am doing on the cover of this book. It is a vigorous pose that we do early in the practice because it requires a lot of strength and builds tremendous fire. I also throw this pose in throughout a class as a way for students to reignite waning energy or heat.

Physically, Crow is based on upper body strength and core power, and learning to balance and be light. But emotionally, it is based on moving through resistance. Crow brings up a lot for people. Some people are afraid of tipping forward onto their heads (which is actually not so bad, since you would only fall a few inches), others come up against extreme frustration because they don't yet have the balance or strength to get into it. For many, it stirs up feelings of competition or perfectionism.

This can be a challenging pose for beginning students, but remember not to get caught up in whether it's hard or easy for you. It doesn't matter. It doesn't matter whether you can do it right away, or whether you are just a baby crow learning to find your wings. What matters is that your spirit is willing and that you are continually working the farthest edge that's healthy for you.

Building Blocks: Setting up the pose correctly is the key to learning Crow. Bring your feet together. Place your hands in front of your feet, flat on the floor, shoulder-width apart. Squat down so your butt hovers a few inches over your heels. Let your elbows and knees drop out laterally, creating a small shelf out of your upper arms. Lean forward and lower your head and chest down a bit. Lift your heels and come up onto your tippy toes, lift your tail high, and rest your knees (or shins) on your upper arms/triceps, near your armpits. Engage a strong abdominal contraction for stability. From there, squeeze your elbows into your torso, press your knees into your arms, and tip your weight for-

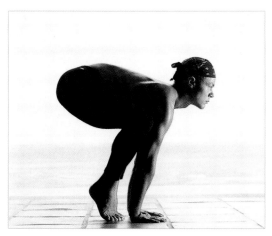

Pose 21: Crow, preparation

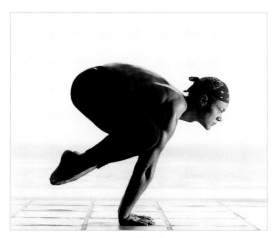

Crow (side)

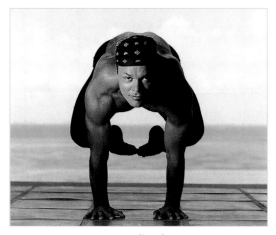

Crow (front)

ward, bringing one foot up off the floor. Gaze at a spot on the floor slightly in front of your hands or, if you can, straight ahead. Take your time to find your balance and then bring the other foot off the floor. If both feet are off the floor, touch your big toes to each other and try to straighten your arms. Remember, equanimity, calm determination, and breathing!

For beginning students, you may only be able to get one foot off the floor, and that's fine. If you can get one foot up, you're a baby crow. Just keep trying and eventually you will take flight!

Alignment:

- Keep the back rounded.
- Contract your abdominal muscles.
- Lift your head and shoulders.
- Straighten your arms as much as you can.
- If both feet are off the floor, touch your big toes together.
- Set a calm, determined gaze forward.

Modification: If you can only bring one foot off the floor, do that. If a fear of falling forward is holding you back, place a pillow or folded blanket on the floor in front of you until you get more comfortable.

Spiritual Focus: Letting go means giving up attachment to results. When you understand that you don't have to try hard, you can give up the fight for results, because you know that ultimately things will work out as they should. Desiring a certain goal in a pose and working to achieve it is different from trying to control the outcome. Just be willing to relax and let go. Know that if one door closes, five new doors will open up. That is true faith: trusting the natural ebb and flow of life.

Connecting Vinyasa

Using your core power, shoot your legs straight back or walk them back to High Push-Up (8) position. Go through Vinyasa A, finishing with Jump Forward (11). Roll up through your spine, sweeping your arms over your head and reaching high, into Mountain pose (5). This sets you up for the next pose, which is Eagle pose.

4. Balancing Series: Equanimity

Balancing poses command our presence. They make us come to center and let go of everything else but the present moment. You don't need to "have good balance" to do these poses. We are all born with a natural sense of balance. All you need is to quiet your mind, focus, and relax. The more you struggle, the more tension you create in your mind and your muscles and the harder it is. The more you relax into these poses, the more things settle in. From there you intuitively create neutral alignment and discover your own weightlessness. You discover that you can stand calm in the eye of any storm.

The two key elements to all balancing postures are breath and focused gaze (drishti). As you already know, your breath brings you into the here and now. It facili-

tates balance because it lets you tune out the distractions and tune in to your body. A concentrated gaze steadies and centers you, streamlining your attention to a single bright beam of energy. This added dimension of a laserlike mind makes every balancing pose a meditation in motion.

Balancing poses tone your lower body, but they also do much more. They balance the left and right sides of your brain, and restore and stabilize your equilibrium.

There are five poses in the balancing series, the first of which (Eagle pose) we do on both the right and left sides. Then we do the next three poses (Standing Leg Raise, Front; Standing Leg Raise, Side; and Airplane) in a flow, first the right side all the way through, then the left side. The fifth, Dancer's Pose, we do on its own four times (right leg, left leg, and repeat).

Pose 22: Eagle Pose (Garudasana)

By standing on one leg, as you do in Eagle pose, you isometrically chisel and tone every muscle in the standing leg and buttock cheek. Eagle pose also opens the hips and shoulders and stretches the upper back. This pose demands your presence and cultivates balance, strength, and serenity.

Building Blocks: With your arms high, exhale and wrap your right arm under the left arm like soft rope, bringing your elbows up to shoulder height. Press your palms together and extend your fingers straight up. Bend your knees to a 45-degree angle

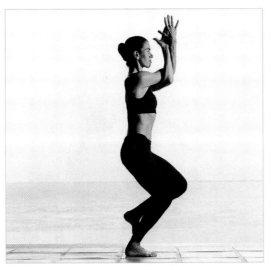

Pose 22: Eagle (side)

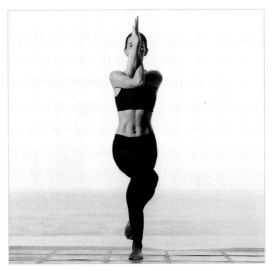

Eagle (front)

and in one fluid motion sweep your right leg up and over the left. If you can, hook your right foot around the bottom of the left calf. Square your hips and chest to the front wall. Your pelvis is tucked under you and your shoulders are stacked directly above your hips. From the side your spine is one straight line. Relax into a center line of gravity. Pull the tops of your shoulders back and down. Set your eyes on a point directly in front of you and breathe through your whole body.

There are three actions at work in Eagle pose: centering your hips and shoulders, opening your chest, and creating spinal length and space. To square your hips, imagine holding a bowl of water on your pelvic floor. Try not to let a single drop spill out over the front edge of your pelvis! Scoop your tailbone in and slightly under and pull the front of your pelvis up toward your abdomen. Draw the pit of the belly in and up. You also want to align your hips horizontally; concentrate on keeping both hip bones level and pointing straight ahead.

It's common to see students wobble, do a little dance on one leg, and then fall out of this pose in the beginning. But the problem isn't that they can't balance, it's that they are struggling rather than surrendering. Use your breath to find your center line of gravity and relax into it. Let go of the strain and struggle. Your body wants to balance. It is coded for this kind of movement if you'll just get your brain out of the way and allow your body to be free.

As with all balancing poses, your gaze is essential. Balance comes from a calm, centered mind. Remember, we set our mind beginning with our eyes. Fix your eyes to one point and take aim. Bring your mind from distraction to direction. Hone in on one point of concentration and you'll become more deeply aware of all points.

Suddenly you really start to see, to hear, to feel like never before.

Hold for five breaths; on the fifth exhalation, dip down a little deeper. Inhale and come sweeping up to standing. Repeat the same instructions in reverse for the left side. We take this pose two times on each side—right, left, right, left—then finish in Samasthiti.

Alignment:

- Bend your standing leg.
- Scoop your tailbone down and under.
- Center your pelvis.
- Raise your elbows high, in line with your shoulders.
- Stack your forearms over your elbows.
- Pull the tops of your shoulders back and down.
- Point your fingers straight up.
- Lift your torso up and dip down into your standing leg.
- Fuse your gaze forward to a set point.

Risk Factor: Be careful not to let the standing knee turn inward. Keep the knee facing forward.

Modification: Set the toes of the raised foot on the floor, to the outside of the standing foot.

Spiritual Focus: Nobility requires no great deed, only relaxed awareness, openness to receive wisdom, and an unwavering alignment to what you feel is right. We learn to soar not through effort but through faith.

Pose 23: Standing Leg Raise, Front (Utthita Hasta Padangusthasana A)

This powerful weight-bearing pose tones and hones the entire standing leg. It also stretches the back side of the raised leg and the muscles between the shoulder blades.

Building Blocks: From Samasthiti, bring your hands together at Namaste and gaze down at your fingertips. Take a moment to find your breath and to access that calm space of serenity within you. When you are ready, bring your gaze forward, taking aim at a fixed spot ahead of you, and place your left hand on your left hip. Then very, very slowly, with as little movement as possible, inhale and squeeze your right knee into your chest with your right hand, keeping your standing leg and spine straight. If you are new to this or your balance is challenged, then stay right here holding your knee. Otherwise, with your left hand still on your left hip, grab your right big toe with the first two fingers of the right hand. Inhale, lengthen the spine, and unhinge your knee to whatever degree you can while still maintaining a straight spine. More important than a straight leg is a straight spine, so if you start to round your back, you know you've gone too far.

Keep your standing leg straight and strong. Engaging your abdominal lock (uddiyana) is very important to stabilize this pose and create weightlessness. Drop your right hip down so it is even with the left—the tendency is to let it roll up. Drop your

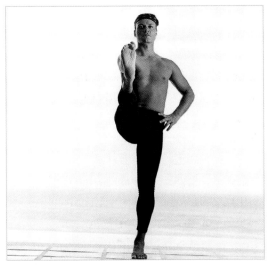

Pose 23: Standing Leg Raise (front)

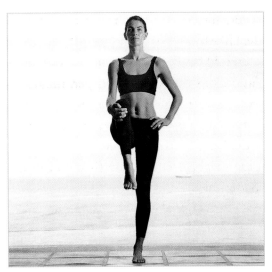

Standing Leg Raise (front), modification

right inner thigh in and down, toward the perineum (the muscle between the anus and genitals). Keep your torso square, your shoulders aligned. Press your shoulders down, away from your ears. Establish your core of gravity and hold for five breaths.

It's OK if you fall, because falling is learning. Your ego hates falling, because it means you've "failed." But your spirit loves falling, because it is a chance to grow and learn as a result. As Lao-tzu taught, success is not found in never falling, but rather in getting up every time we fall.

Hold for five breaths, then flow right into the next pose, which is Standing Leg Raise, Side.

Alignment:
- Body stature is upright and extended, as in Samasthiti.
- Maintain a straight spine and contract your belly inward.

- Keep your standing leg strong and straight.
- Keep both buttocks and hips level to the floor.
- Rotate the inner thigh of the standing leg back toward the back wall.
- Keep your shoulders on one plane; do not turn your torso.
- Gaze forward at a single point.

Risk Factor: Rounding your back to straighten the leg strains the lower and middle back.

Modification: Keep your upper knee bent. You can also lean against a wall.

Spiritual Focus: When we come out of our head stuff—the mental systems and thought patterns that say we can't or won't—we suddenly realize the ways we are limiting ourselves. Just for the moment, forget what you believe you can't do. The on-the-mat truth is that very often our body is stronger and more flexible than our faith.

Pose 24: Standing Leg Raise, Side (Utthita Hasta Padangusthasana B)

This pose is similar to Standing Leg Raise, Front, and has much of the same transformational effects. In addition, it is a powerful force in opening and strengthening the hip and pelvic muscles.

Building Blocks: From Standing Leg Raise, Front, open your right leg (if you are holding your toe) or your knee (if you are holding your knee) out to the right side. Then turn your head so your gaze is to the left wall. Drop your right hip down in line with the left. Keep that straight line in your spine; bend your knee slightly if necessary to maintain spinal integrity. Every-thing else stays the same as the previous pose.

The tendency is to try to bring the leg way up, but it's really more about bringing it out to the side than up. Flexibility and vertical lift will come in time; what you want to work here is the centering and opening of the right hip. Keep your hips level; don't let the right hip come up. Again, rotate the inner thigh of the raised leg up, toward the ceiling.

Alignment:

Same as for Standing Leg Raise, Front, plus:

- Drop your right hip down in line with your left.
- Set your eyes over your left shoulder.

Risk Factor: Pulling the leg up too high takes your hips off line and disrupts your balance.

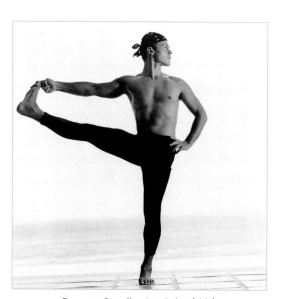

Pose 24: Standing Leg Raise (side)

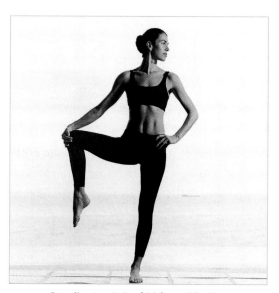

Standing Leg Raise (side), modification

Modification: Work with the upper knee bent or use a belt to catch the foot. If you need help with balance you can extend your free arm straight out to the left, like a wing.

Spiritual Focus: One of the principles of yoga is not to seek the fruits of your actions. Practice for its own sake, without regard to success or failure. This is the way to equanimity.

Connecting Vinyasa

Bring the extended leg and gaze back to center. Release the toe (or knee) and place your hands on your hips. Extend the leg out straight and take five full breaths. Then bend your right knee. This will lead you right into the next posture, Airplane pose.

Pose 25: Airplane Pose (Dekasana)

Airplane is another one-leg balancing pose that tones the entire standing leg and cultivates overall flexible strength and lightness. Using every muscle of the body, it stabilizes and integrates the torso, hips, and legs by hovering on a new plane of gravity. As with all the poses in this series, the balance comes from a quiet, centered mind. You may feel a little unstable at first, but if you stay calm you will find the confidence you need. Know, without a shadow of a doubt, that you can do this. Believe it. Just be light and fly above it all.

Building Blocks: Standing upright, still balancing on one leg, bring your hands to your hips and your right knee in to your chest. In one liquid motion, exhale, hinge forward and extend your right leg out behind you. Your torso and upper leg should be parallel to the floor. Drop your right hip down, then spiral your right inner thigh up to the sky. Open your arms out behind you like wings, with your palms facing down. Draw your shoulder blades down your back and together. Your torso is hovering forward, but your chest is slightly higher than your hips. Arch your back very slightly, as though you were bringing a little Upward Facing Dog into this movement. Lower your chin so your neck is in a neutral position and gaze at the floor about two feet in front of your standing foot. Be light and free in mind and body.

There are five active lines of energy in the Airplane pose, each radiating like a five-point star: two arms, two legs, and the torso. The standing leg presses down into the floor, the inner wall of your chest pulls forward and away from the pelvis, and your arms and raised leg extend back and away from the epicenter of your body. Be aware of all five points at all times and continually work full expression through them.

Alignment:
- Squeeze your legs and root down through the standing foot.
- Spiral the inner thigh of the raised leg upward and the outer thigh downward.
- Keep your upper foot active.
- Square your hips to the floor.
- Stretch the wall of your chest forward, creating traction through your torso.

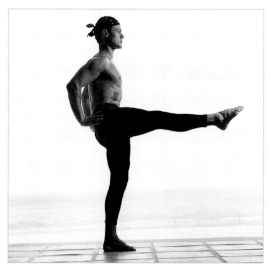

Pose 25: Airplane, preparation

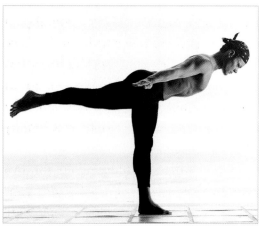

Airplane

- Draw your shoulder blades down your back.
- Pull your arms back and radiate through the fingertips.
- Gaze at the floor about two feet in front of your standing foot.

Risk Factor: Beware of hyperextending the standing knee. Keep the leg straight but not locked. Don't round your back forward—this strains the spine. Also, do not wobble on the standing ankle; keep it stable.

Modification: Bring your torso forward to an angle that is comfortable for you. You can also soften the standing knee slightly.

Spiritual Focus: Mental surrender combined with calm determination makes us open and receptive to change. Through surrender we suddenly tap a supportive inner force and life-giving energy that sustains us and propels us forward and upward. Let go, fasten your spiritual seat belt, and take flight!

Connecting Vinyasa

From Airplane pose, lower the raised leg and very slowly come rolling back up to standing with a strong sense of torso stabilization. Bring your hands up to Namaste at your heart center on the exhale and once again repeat the sequence of these three poses (Standing Leg Raise, Front; Standing Leg Raise, Side; and Airplane), this time on the left side. End in Samasthiti.

Pose 26: Dancer's Pose (Natarajasana)

Dancer's Pose shows you how to ground and stabilize the legs and gain a greater degree of balance and poise. It ultimately teaches you that the real stretch is always spiritual.

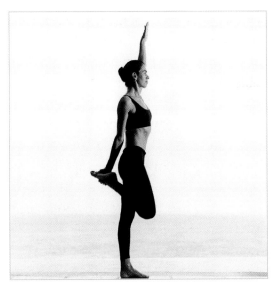

Pose 26: Dancer's Pose, preparation

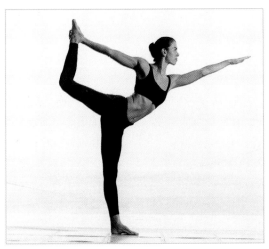

Dancer's Pose

Building Blocks: From standing, bring your left arm up to the sky and roll your right hand open so your palm is facing forward. Bend your right knee and bring your right foot up from behind. Reach your right hand back and grab the inside of your right foot with your thumb pointing up

like a hitchhiker. Bring your knees together. Set your gaze and take a moment to establish your balance and dial into your center line of gravity. When your foundation feels stable, inhale, lift your heart center high, and then stretch forward. Keep your chest up a little higher than your hips. Reach your left shoulder forward and right leg back. Extend and straighten the back leg as much as you can.

This pose translates to "standing bow." You want to create a strong tension between your back leg and your upper body, as if your legs are the bow and your torso the arrow. The back leg is resisting the torso's pull forward. You should feel as if you are hanging from the back leg. The back leg is active, the torso free and suspended. Be conscious not to let your raised hip roll up to an extreme; the upper hip does lift, but only to a healthy degree.

Never stop breathing! Hold for five breaths, then release and helicopter your arms so your right arm is up. Repeat these steps for the left side. Do the pose once more on the right and once more on the left, ending in Samasthiti (4).

Alignment:
- Maintain a strong action in the legs as the "bow."
- Launch your upper body forward, like an arrow.
- Extend your front arm and reach endlessly forward through your fingertips.

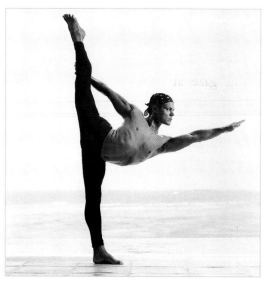

Dancer's Pose, full extension

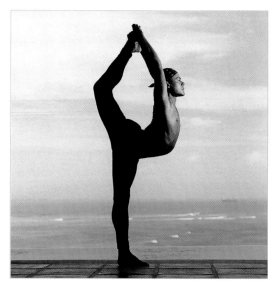

Full Bow

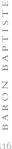
- Spread and stretch the muscles and tendons in your chest and shoulders.
- Set a soft, steady, and determined gaze forward.

Risk Factor: Beware of hyperextending the standing knee. You need to work with your leg straight but not locked. Don't jam your neck upward or force the stretch into your lower back.

Spiritual Focus: The goal of this practice is to find a pace and intensity that is most appropriate for us "Try easy" is a reminder that, in terms of our growth, it is not a good idea for us to move ahead too quickly. As we become gentler with ourselves, it becomes natural for us to have a deeper compassion for others and to live with true grace.

Pose 27: Tree Pose (Vrksasana)

After all the heat and strength built up through the vinyasa up to this point, this pose brings you into a natural state of stillness in both mind and body. This pose is an extension of a seated meditation. It has an eternal quality because once you lock into the position, it holds itself and you feel as if you could stay there effortlessly forever. That is the meditative state.

However peaceful Tree pose may be, it is definitely not a resting pose. In fact, it uses all the elements we have built up until now. It elevates your healing heat, balance, and lower body strength to a whole other level.

Building Blocks:

Step one: From Samasthiti, lift your left heel high and place the sole of your left breath and focused gaze to steady yourself. Bring your hands to Namaste at your heart center and gaze forward (to deepen your focus, gaze at your fingertips). Pressing your palms together will help stabilize you. Hold for five breaths.

Step two: Release your hands and sweep your arms up over your head, palms facing each other. Interlace your fingers and spin your wrists so your palms face up. Move your elbows in toward each other. Extend your spine and reach up. Be of heaven and earth. Like a tree, extend your roots down and blossom your arms up toward the sun. The stronger the roots, the taller the tree.

Your standing leg needs to be powerfully engaged to support you in this pose. Squeeze your left buttock and lift and contract your quadricep. Your hips should be even, even if that means bringing your raised leg forward a bit. Conjure up the image of your pelvis as a water bowl and do not let the water flow over the front edge.

Breathe free and easy. Stand tall and relax into a standing meditation. Let go of your thoughts and just come into your breath and your body. On the fifth exhalation, release your hands and return to Samasthiti. Repeat on the right side, ending in Samasthiti.

Alignment:
• Maintain one central line of energy through your entire body.

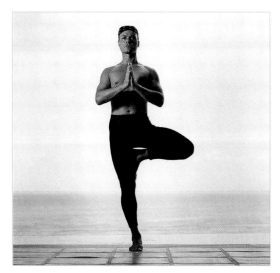

Pose 27: Tree

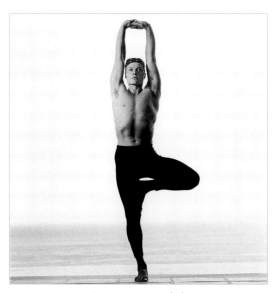

Tree, arms extended

foot onto your inner right thigh. Be mindful of your knee—never wrench! Press down through the sole of your right foot, really taking the time to establish your balance on your standing leg. Drop your left hip down in line with the right. Use your

- Center your hips (both front to back and side to side).
- Gently lift and contract your abdominal core.
- Stretch the sides of your waist upward to your fingertips.
- Elongate your spine.
- Squeeze your elbows in toward each other.
- Relax your face, neck, and throat.
- Relax your eyes forward, toward the horizon.

Risk Factor: Be mindful not to lock and/or hyperextend the standing knee joint. Do not arch your back or push your rib cage forward.

Modification: If it is difficult to balance, lower your foot to a point on the standing leg that is comfortable.

Spiritual Focus: The only trees that survive hurricanes are the ones that have deep roots and the supple strength to bend with the storm winds. Equanimity allows you to stand tall and secure no matter what storms life brings your way.

Connecting Vinyasa

Release your hands and foot and come back to Samasthiti. Repeat Tree pose on the other side. Release, ending in Samasthiti. Then go through Vinyasa B to Warrior I (13), then into Warrior II (14). This sets you in position for the next pose, Triangle.

5. Triangle Series: Grounding

The poses in the Triangle Series work your whole body into a beautiful symmetrical stability and poise. They increase strength in the legs, hips, and back, which gives you a sense of overall balance, body confidence, and courage. Your lower body is your ground of being and your connection to the earth. Strengthening from the waist down enables you to create deep, penetrating roots from which you can blossom and open your body straight up to the sun.

There are four poses in the Triangle Series: Triangle, Twisting Triangle, Standing Straddle Bend, and Namaste Forward Bend. The first two are done as a flow, right side first the whole way through, then left side the whole way through. The third and fourth poses are done in completion on their own, with connecting vinyasa in between.

Pose 28: Triangle Pose (Trikonasana)

Triangle is a beautiful pose that sends life through your whole body. It gives you the opportunity to seek out and fill any deflated or compressed kinks in your body. Here you can work your breath and lines of energy to fill out the contours of your pose. It sculpts the legs, hips, and butt and creates an overall opening through your chest and back.

Building Blocks: From Warrior II, first check your alignment and make sure your front

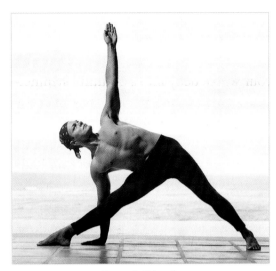

Pose 28: Triangle

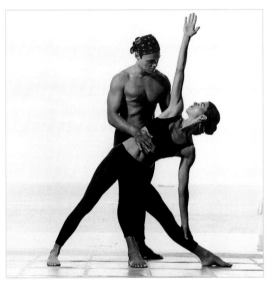

Triangle, modification

toward the ankle and eventually to the floor). Bring your left arm up to the sky. Your arms should be stacked in one vertical line. Resist the temptation to sit in the lower shoulder; you want to lift up out of it and create full extension from fingertip to fingertip. Draw your scapulae down toward your hips.

Your legs should be straight and powerful. Engage your upper thighs as you spin your inner thighs outward and away from each other. Pull your tail and belly in. Your torso should be stacked over your right thigh. Meditate on your left thumbnail.

You want your entire body—your hips, head, and heart—all on one plane, as if you are standing perfectly centered between two panes of glass. A common mistake in Triangle pose is to roll the upper shoulder downward toward the floor, which rotates your torso down and potentially puts your joint system at risk. You want to really focus on dropping the lower side of your rib cage toward the floor, stacking your upper lung over the lower, so your chest is open to the side wall. This will keep your torso rotating up and give you full expression through your whole upper body.

Alignment:
- Heels are in one line.
- Maintain strong action through the legs.
- Spiral your inner thighs outward, away from each other.
- Scoop your tailbone down and under.
- Radiate through both arms.
- Keep your upper hand active.

knee is stacked over your ankle. As you inhale, straighten your front knee on the same plane as your foot and tilt your tailbone/pelvis to the back wall, as you reach your right arm forward. Reach down and grab your right shin (if this is easy to accomplish, you can lower your hand down

- Lift the pit of your belly inward to lengthen your spine.
- Drop your lower rib cage toward the floor.
- Twist your torso, stacking your upper lung over your lower lung.
- Draw your scapulae down toward your hips.
- Gaze high to your upper thumbnail.

Modification: If it is difficult to keep your torso stacked over your thigh, bring your hand higher up on your shin, or to your thigh. You can also use a block under your lower hand. Gaze down if looking up strains your neck.

Spiritual Focus: When you sculpt with clay, you have to keep it moist so that it stays malleable. You have to spray it with water, otherwise it will dry out and harden. Our relaxed mind is to the body what water is to clay. As the mind relaxes, so will your body. With each breath, let go a little more. Be fluid . . . relax, breathe, and flow.

Connecting Vinyasa

After five full breaths, inhale and let your raised arm pull you up to standing. From here you'll flow right into the next pose, Twisting Triangle.

Pose 29: Twisting Triangle (Parivrtta Trikonasana)

This is a deep twisting pose that squeezes and rinses all the organs and tissue of your mid-body, including your digestive system. It wrings out toxins from the liver, spleen, colon, gallbladder, and kidneys and releases the lumbar spine and helps relieve lower back pain. Twisting Triangle coordinates your whole body into one unified force.

Building Blocks: From Triangle pose, bring your hands to your hips and square them to the wall in front of you. You'll probably need to turn your back foot in to a 45-degree angle in order to do this. Step your back foot in a little, bringing your feet about three to four feet apart. Really take the time to center your hips, because they will be your anchor in this pose.

Bring your left arm up next to your ear. As you inhale, reach way up high through your left hand (creating length through your spine) and on the exhalation, hinge forward from your hips and place the left palm on the floor to the outside of your right foot (or to the right leg, shin, foot, or on a block—wherever feels stable). Engage your abdominal lock. Use your hand to pull your right hip back in line with your left. Inhale, roll the right shoulder back, and extend the right arm straight up as you exhale. It's okay if your back heel comes off the floor a little bit. Press through both arms, which should be on one vertical line. Stretch your chest toward your chin and your butt backward. As with regular Triangle pose, draw your scapulae down your back toward your hips. Turn your head and set your eyes high to your upper thumbnail.

It is essential to work toward a straight

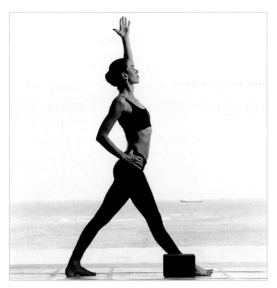

Pose 29: Twisting Triangle, preparation

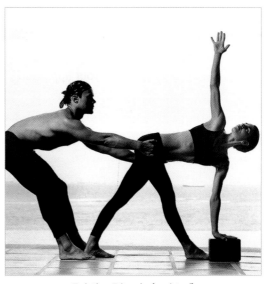

Twisting Triangle (assisted)

spine in Twisting Triangle; you never want to twist with a round back. So continually extend and lengthen your spine on every inhalation and work the rotation on the exhalations. Don't force the twist! Simply revolve around as far as is healthy for you and work the pose there.

You want to really engage your legs as the foundation in this pose. The stronger your lower body, the more extension you will have through the upper half. It's also important to focus on twisting from the torso, not the shoulders. Pull your right hip back, your left hip forward, working your legs like a pair of scissors. Turn your hips like a steering wheel until your pelvis is squared.

There is a balancing element to Twisting Triangle, so as with all balancing poses, set your gaze on one spot and breathe through that concentrated vision.

Alignment:

- Square your hips forward.
- Engage powerful legs!
- Bring your inner thighs together.
- Lift the pit of your belly and work a straight line through your spine.
- On the inhalation, elongate your spine. On the exhalation, twist.
- Initiate the twist from your hips and torso.
- Press your sitting bones back away from your head.
- Stack your torso over your front leg.
- Twist your torso upward, using your abdominal lock and your hips as a steering wheel.
- Drop your shoulder blades toward your hips and spread them apart.
- Line up your arms along a vertical plane and reach through the upper fingertips.
- Relax your face.

- Gaze high through your upper hand (or down at the floor, if that feels better on your neck).

Risk Factor: Twisting too far past your edge strains the middle and lower back and the spine. Just be true to yourself and pay attention to what your body needs. Also, you never want to rotate a rounded back—it causes compression. Always extend your spine before you twist.

Modification: If you have a block, you can place it to the outside of your front foot and rest your hand on it. You can also lift your back heel; this will allow you to work with your pelvis, centering it and getting more leverage in your twist.

Spiritual Focus: Becoming impatient and frustrated with ourselves is our way of trying to control the outcomes of what we're doing. Our willingness to relax, breathe, and stay calm and in the moment allows us to discover what is possible. When we relax, we align ourselves with a power and energy that ultimately works on our behalf in all dimensions of our lives.

Connecting Vinyasa

From Twisting Triangle, look down toward the floor and helicopter your arms up to standing. Step your back foot forward to Samasthiti and go through Vinyasa B again, this time stepping into Warrior I with your left foot. Repeat the previous sequence of Triangle (26) and Twisting Triangle (27) with your left foot forward. From your second Twisting Triangle, helicopter your arms up to standing so you are facing the side wall. This puts you in position for the next pose, Standing Straddle Bend.

Pose 30: Standing Straddle Bend (Prasarita Padottanasana A)

This deep hamstring and calf stretch is a great countermovement to any sports training that shortens and tightens the hamstrings, like running or cycling. Inverted forward bends tone the internal organs—the liver, spleen, kidneys, digestive organs, pancreas, and gallbladder. The deep release and introspective quality of this pose also quiets and soothes the nervous system.

Building Blocks: Facing the side wall, toe/heel your feet out so your legs are approximately four to five feet apart. Turn your toes in a little so your feet are slightly pigeon-toed. Catch your hips with your hands and, on the inhalation, lift your chest and chin upward, bringing a slight arch to your back. On the exhalation, hinge forward from your hips and set your hands flat on the floor, shoulder-width apart. Walk your fingers back so they are in line with your toes (eventually with your heels). Inhale, lift halfway up to a flat back with your chest forward and butt back, then exhale and fold forward again. Press your palms into your mat. Bring the crown of your head down as close to the floor as

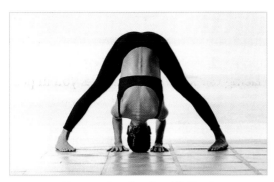

Pose 30: Standing Straddle Bend

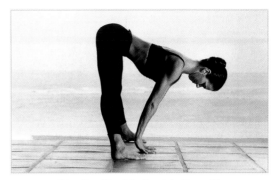

Standing Straddle Bend, halfway lift

you can. Draw your elbows in toward each other to open the back, and use your arms to leverage your stretch. Eventually your arms should be at right angles with the elbows stacked over the wrists.

Sway your hips forward in line with your heels to help release the lower back. Engage your quads, lifting up from the kneecaps. Lift your sitting bones and hamstrings to the heavens. Your legs should be straight and strong. Lift the inner anklebones a bit and press through the outer edges of your feet. Lift your inner thighs away from each other. You want to really open your groin in this pose. You've got good heat inside you now, so the tissue is nice and malleable. Why not use this opportunity to go into new territories of tissue, new frontiers, new thresholds? That's what transformation is all about.

The ideal is to be able to rest the crown of your head on the floor, so with every inhalation extend your spine, and on every exhalation draw the top of your head down. (If your head easily reaches the floor, then shorten the width of your stance.) Now really reach . . . the only thing standing between your head and the floor is your mind!

Alignment:

- Feet are three to five feet apart and parallel.
- Lift your inner anklebones and press into the outer edges of your feet.
- Legs are strong: quads engaged and pulling up from the kneecaps, hamstrings stretched upward, inner thighs pressing away from each other.
- Sway your hips forward in line with your heels.
- Lift your sitting bones and spread them away from each other.
- Press your palms into the mat at shoulder width, fingers in line with your toes (or heels, if you can).
- Rotate your elbows in until shoulder-width apart and use them to spread your shoulder blades apart and broaden your upper back.
- Adjust the weight distribution between the feet, hands, and head from moment to moment. Keep your eyes soft and steady, your face relaxed and free.

Risk Factor: Beware of hyperextending your knees. Keep them straight but not locked. Also, don't sag into your shoulders.

Modification: You can bend your knees or play with the width of your feet to find the perfect pose for your body.

Spiritual Focus: Be aware of all the times in your practice or in a pose when your mind asks, am I doing it right? Is this what I should be feeling? I don't look like the photo in the book—I must be doing it wrong. Doubt these doubts! Let them pass and anchor your mind more deeply in the present moment. Allow this moment to flow into the next without doubting, comparing, judging, or analyzing. Simply observe, be open, accept, embrace what is right here, right now. Only this pose, only this moment.

Connecting Vinyasa

On the inhalation, lift halfway up, gazing forward. On the exhalation, bring your hands to your hips. Inhale and use your abdominal muscles to pull you back up to standing. Inhale. Exhale and open your arms up and out to the sides. Broaden your chest. You are now in position for the next pose, Namaste Forward Bend.

Pose 31: Namaste Forward Bend (Parsvottanasana)

This is an intense stretch that gets way down deep into the hamstrings. It also stretches the front of the shoulders and

chest, and, as in all forward bends, releases all the muscles in the back. Lastly, the reverse Namaste hand position strengthens the wrists, which can be powerfully transformative and therapeutic for conditions like carpal tunnel syndrome and general wrist weaknesses. Strong wrists will help in Downward Facing Dog and ultimately handstands as you continue on in your practice.

Building Blocks: With your arms out to the sides, bring your hands together to what is called "reverse Namaste" at your back. To do this, bring your arms around behind your back to the space between your shoulder blades. Press your palms together in a prayerlike position with the fingers facing up (or down, if up strains your wrists). If your upper body is tight, try grabbing opposite hand to opposite elbow.

Pivot your body to the right so you are

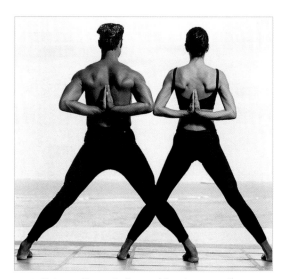

Pose 31: Namaste Forward Bend, preparation

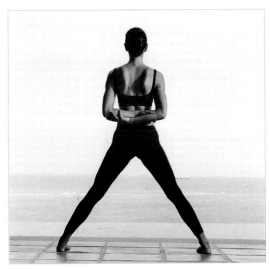

Namaste Forward Bend, preparation modification

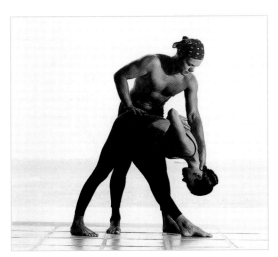

Namaste Forward Bend (assisted)

are in one line. Relax your head and neck and breathe deep.

You'll need to keep your legs strong to maintain your balance in this pose. The back leg must be perfectly straight, but the front knee can soften if you need to decrease the intensity a little. Breathe love into your hamstrings and melt away any tightness or tension that's still there.

Squeeze your shoulder blades in toward each other, lifting your elbows. Press the palms of your hands together. Look to the big toe of your back foot and make it glow with the intensity of your gaze.

Alignment:

- Position your feet three and a half feet apart.
- Maintain a strong and straight back leg.
- Bring your inner thighs together.
- Press the front thigh and sitting bones back.
- Turn your hips like a steering wheel.
- Flirt with the distribution of weight between the legs.
- Keep your hips and shoulders squared.
- Set your belly button over your front thigh.
- With your palms together, lift your elbows away from your back.
- Extend the crown of your head down toward your front foot.
- Allow your head to hang, keeping your neck relaxed and your forehead on your shin.
- Relax every muscle in your forehead and face.

facing the back wall. Open your right foot and step your back foot in a little. Take a moment to square your hips and chest so your hipbones and nipples shine straight ahead. On the inhalation, root down into your legs and lift your chin and chest up, bringing a slight arch to your back. On the exhalation, hinge forward over your front leg. Pull your front hip back so your hips

It is natural to get dizzy in this pose, but the dizziness will pass. It is just stuck energy and toxicity coming up for release. Welcome it and work with it, because if it doesn't come up and out, it stays there! If you get dizzy, do NOT close your eyes—you'll end up a blob on the floor. Keep them open, stay alert, and remember to breathe. If you need to, come down into Child's Pose to regain your equilibrium.

Modification: If the reverse Namaste hurts your wrists, turn your hands so your fingers are facing down. If this is still too intense, hold opposite hand to opposite elbow.

Spiritual Focus: Focus is the key. Take your pose seriously, but take yourself lightly.

Connecting Vinyasa

After five breaths, contract your abdominal muscles, stabilize your torso, and, leading with your chest, use these muscles to pull back up to standing. Keeping your hands in reverse Namaste, pivot on your heels 180 degrees so your left foot is forward. Repeat Namaste Forward Bend on this side for five breaths, then drop your hands to the floor on either side of your front foot, shoulder-width apart. Step your front leg back and come into the High Push-Up (8) position. From there, go to Low Push-Up (9) and then Upward Facing Dog (10). This puts you in position for the next pose, Locust.

6. Backbending Series: Igniting

When people age they tend to contract and pull into themselves. But yoga, and especially the spinal work we do in yoga, can actually reverse the aging process. You are only as young as your spine is supple, and these poses are the best way to keep your spine limber. If you are tight or weak in any part of your back, backbends are like medicine. Your energy system is centralized along your spine, and backbends remove blocks of energy stored there. They ignite electricity in your spine and bring your whole being to a healthier realm.

We live our lives in a forward direction. For the most part we walk, sit, drive, reach, communicate, and live in one direction. At the same time, gravity pulls us downward. Going backward generates awesome elasticity and suppleness in the hips. Backbends strengthen and sculpt the entire back while simultaneously creating true structural integrity. They empower and strengthen while dissolving heaviness of the heart and dullness of the mind.

Moving back requires courage and a sense of adventure as we move into the unfamiliar and unknown territory of what lies behind us. For many people, there is a fear that accompanies going backward. We are exposing our soft body (the abdomen and internal organs), which makes us feel vulnerable. This can bring up emotions that have been hidden in unknown places within us, allowing them to surface for release. Symbolically, going backward may represent returning to your past. But sometimes we need to go back in order to go forward, both physically and emotionally.

In all backbending poses, it is very important that you stay alert and conscious to what you are doing. Almost all injuries result when someone is not fully present. If you've ever been in an accident, you know it's usually because someone wasn't paying attention, even if only for a split second. Please, stay centered, *stay focused,* and stay in your body and breathe when doing backbends.

The Backbending Series consists of five poses (Locust, Bow, Camel, Bridge, and Wheel) and one neutralizing pose (Supta Baddha Konasana).

Pose 32: Locust (Salabhasana)

As the first pose in the spinal series, Locust brings your awareness to the spine and flushes the whole back side with fresh blood. You can feel the warmth bathe your whole body when you come out of this pose. It also lengthens and opens the front of the body and gives the digestive and other vital organs a deep and powerful massage. Locust conditions, hones, and creates a stabilizing strength in every muscle on the back side of the body, including the buttocks and thighs. It relaxes and eliminates tension, aches, and pains in the back.

Building Blocks: After holding Upward Facing Dog for five breaths, roll over your

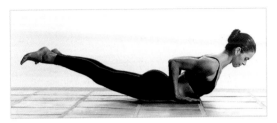

Pose 32: Locust

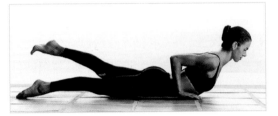

Locust, modification

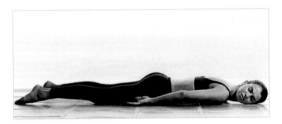

Rest from Locust (and Bow)

toes and go back into Downward Facing Dog for five breaths. From here, come forward into High Push-Up, and breathe in and out. To the count of five, lower yourself all the way to the floor. Rest on your mat and relax for a moment. Rest your arms by your side, palms facing up, and lay your head to one side. Love the floor like never before! Your practice opens you up to be grateful for all things . . . even a hard floor.

You may need to pad your hipbones here. You can use a towel or just fold up your mat. Flip your palms down to the floor and bring them in line with your hips, fingers facing forward, elbows bent and tucked into your sides. Bring your chin to the floor. Separate your feet so your legs are hip-width apart. Inhale, and in one fluid motion, lift your chest, ribs, thighs, and feet up off the floor. Ideally you want nothing but your palms, pelvis, and lower belly touching the floor. Squeeze your butt and thighs! Your legs must be straight and active, funneling energy through the balls of your feet. Spin your inner thighs up to the sky. Your feet are either together or hip-width apart.

Pull your heart muscle forward. Lower your head so your neck is long and in line with your spine. The crown of your head should be facing forward (men, the bald spot on the top of your head should be shining on the wall in front of you). Reach long, with full-body extension. Focus on the forward and backward action of your body—a tug-of-war. On the in breath the chest swells forward, on the out breath the legs extend back and up, as though someone was behind you pulling them out of your hip sockets. After five breaths, relax down, bringing one cheek to one side. Repeat this pose twice, ending with your cheek to the other side on your mat.

Alignment:

- Set your hands alongside your hips.
- Squeeze your butt and thighs.
- Legs are hip-width apart or together.
- Spiral your inner thighs up to the ceiling.
- Press your tailbone to the floor.
- Create traction from the balls of your feet through the crown of your head.
- Drop your shoulder blades down toward your hips.
- Draw your elbows into your ribs and pull the mat back with your hands.
- Keep your head down, your neck neutral, free, and relaxed.
- Drop your mask and soften your eyes.

Risk Factor: You can strain your neck by jamming your chin up. Also, take care not to strain your lower back.

Modification: If this pose bothers your lower back, just bring one leg up at a time. Do the right leg and then the left.

Spiritual Focus: The present moment is forever new and offers a fresh beginning. In this moment our minds can be made new. In this moment our bodies can be electrified and made new. Not through suffering and pain, but through a new perception. Rewire your mind right here, right now, in this one moment and your whole world can change.

Pose 33: Bow Pose (Dhanurasana)

The Bow pose continues the stimulating effects of backbends and further strengthens and conditions the back side of the body. It is also an amazing chest-opener and a profound release for the fronts of the shoulders, hips, and thighs. Balancing your weight on your mid-body is like a tremendous massage for the digestive organs. The healthy pressure stimulates the kidneys and adrenals.

Building Blocks: From the resting position after Locust, bring your chin back to the floor. Bend your knees and bring them to hip width. Lift your heels up. Reach back with both arms and grab the tops of your feet with your thumbs pointing toward the floor (or, to deepen it, hold the outsides of your ankles and flex your feet). On the inhalation, press back through your legs as you lift your thighs and chest off the floor and pull your torso forward. Your legs are the anchor from which you are suspending your torso's weight. The legs are resisting, the torso relaxing. This is the same forward-and-back action you took in Dancer's Pose (which is the standing bow pose). The tighter the bow, the more spring you get for the arrow. Use your breath to lift both ends up. The complete expression of this pose is when you are extending your arms and legs straight up, forming an apex with your hands and feet.

Drop your head forward and relax your neck. Breathe through any tension. Spread your toes and keep them animated. Really relax into the pose—be as strain-free as you can be. After five breaths, relax down and rest with one cheek to one side. Repeat this pose a second time, relaxing down,

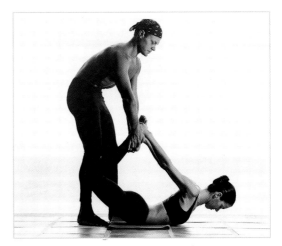

Pose 33: Bow (assisted)

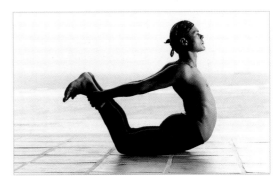

Bow

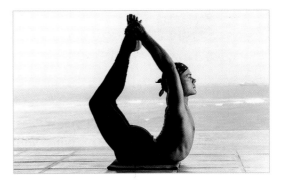

Full Bow

with the other cheek against your mat. Then come into Down Dog (2) for a little rest and rejuvenation.

Alignment:

- Activate your feet and spread your toes.
- Spread your knees to hip width.
- Spiral your inner thighs to the ceiling.
- Maintain very strong legs as your anchor.
- Press your tailbone down toward the floor.
- Your legs move back, your chest moves forward, then everything moves up.
- Lower body active, upper body relaxed and suspended.
- Drop your head forward and let the neck muscles stretch.
- Soften your mask and gaze gently at one point on the floor.

Risk Factor: Beware of letting your knees splay out wider than hip width. This puts the lower body joint systems at risk. Also, cranking your chin up can strain your neck.

Modification: If this hurts your lower back, bring one leg up at a time.

Spiritual Focus: The idea of relaxing, doing less, and going with the flow can scare us. We feel that we are hardly measuring up and doing enough as it is. We say to ourselves, "If I do less and become more passive I'll never achieve anything." But a relaxed energy has its own kind of power. Our personal force is strongest when we balance action with relaxation, like a bow and arrow. The bow provides tension from which the arrow releases. Neither is as effective without the energy of the other, and combined they carry you forward with astonishing power and grace.

Pose 34: Camel (Ustrasana)

Camel pose is the reverse position of sitting. Sitting is demanding and not a resting position. A consistent sitter is slowly bent out of shape and usually lacks the structural support and strength to sit in neutral, symmetrical, and natural alignment. Thus the back, neck, and shoulders all suffer. The front side of the torso and hips tighten, and over time the chest collapses forward, causing the shoulders to tighten as well. Just like an athlete in training, the professional sitter has created body imbalances and potential injury.

Backbending poses like Camel can help undo this. It is a terrific hip opener that releases the muscles you use for sitting. It releases the hip flexors, psoas, and some of the rotator muscles, which affect the entire body's ability to move, whether in sports or in everyday life. It stretches and opens the entire front side of the torso (chest, abdominal wall, pectoral minor muscles, front of the shoulders, and biceps). You will also find a powerful emotional dimension to this pose that opens your heart center and sparks the emotional center of your body.

Building Blocks: From Downward Dog, come onto your knees with your shins pressing into the floor. You may want to double the mat under your knees for a little extra padding. Separate your knees and feet until they are hip-width apart. Bring your hands to your lower back with your fingers pointing up, thumbs into your

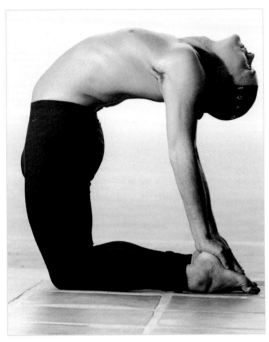

Pose 34: Camel

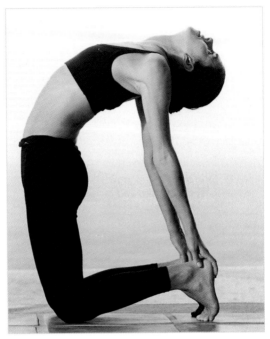

Camel, modification

sacrum, and contract the muscles in your lower body. Your lower body needs to be very strong in this pose; the power in back-bending poses comes from leg strength. Find your breath. Set your eyes, exhale, and scoop your tailbone down and under, then inhale your chest up and gently release your head back as a natural expression of a full backbend. Be careful with your neck. If this feels comfortable, reach back and set a hand on each heel, one at a time. **Scooping your tailbone under first is very important to protect your lower back!** The palms of your hands should be cupping your heels with your thumbs to the outside of your ankles. (If this feels difficult, see the modification.)

Really squeeze from the waist down—

your butt, thighs, and hamstrings contracting. From that strength, breathe as you energetically lift your chest toward the sky. Root down and lift up. Press your shinbones down with force and raise your heart high! Your chest lifts up, up, up, your heart center opens and expands like a helium balloon. You are not resting your upper body weight on your arms so much as your arms are like a taut line tied to your heels, preventing your chest wall from rocketing straight up through the ceiling. Press your hips forward a little. Move your shoulder blades down your back, pressing them away from your ears. You should feel a terrific stretch in your upper trapezium muscles (the muscles between your neck and shoulders).

After five breaths, tuck your chin to your

chest, squeeze your lower body and root down, and from that leg strength slowly float back up to standing on your shins. Relax back down into Child's Pose (or to keep the heat up, take Downward Facing Dog). Repeat Camel pose once more, going just a little bit farther the second time. Then go to Down Dog, take a few breaths, and rest in Child's Pose.

Alignment:

- Root the shins, ankles, and feet down into the floor.
- Scoop your tailbone under and pull the front of your pelvis upward.
- Engage your abdominal lock.
- Engage your lower body, making it very strong.
- Press your hips forward until the thighs are vertical.
- Lift your chest up.
- Drop your shoulder blades down your back.
- Release your head back.
- Fill out the full shape and expression of your body.
- Soften your face and set your eyes on the wall behind you.

Risk Factor: Dropping your head back can strain your neck if it's tight, so pay close attention to what it needs. One way to protect your neck (and also to prevent blocking your airways) in all backbends is to first tuck your chin down and back slightly, as though you were holding a pencil under your chin, and then slowly drop your head back. Or simply work the pose with your head up and your chin to your chest.

Modification: If your lower back is tight, you can come up onto the balls of your feet—this will dilute the intensity of the movement by 40 percent. To dilute it even further, keep your hands at your low back, fingers facing up and pressing your sitting muscles down, then bend backward to a comfortable degree.

Spiritual Focus: The human body is a masterpiece of ingenuity. Without us having to think about it, our hearts beat about 100,000 times a day, our lungs expand and contract, and our body constantly re-creates itself. In a challenging moment, we should trust its brilliance. Instead of telling it what to do or how far to go, let it tell you. Trust that small, quiet, secret voice—it knows!

Connecting Vinyasa

From Child's Pose, reach your arms forward and step your feet back, coming into Downward Facing Dog (2). (If you are already in Downward Facing Dog, stay there.) Take active rest in Downward Facing Dog for a few breaths, then look forward to your hands, bend your knees, and jump through your arms to sitting. No big deal here, just do the best you can to jump forward to a cross-legged position. (If you prefer, walk your feet up to your hands and then sit.) Move back a little on your mat and lie on your back. You are now in position for the next pose, Bridge.

Pose 35: Bridge Pose (Setu Bandhasana)

Bridge pose has many benefits: It opens the chest and stretches the abdominal wall; tones the butt and thighs; and stabilizes, releases, and brings relief to the lower back. It opens the breathing body, creating a new awareness and rhythm.

Building Blocks: Lie on your back and place your feet flat on the floor hip-width apart, knees over your heels (*not* the toes). Tilt your pelvis and scoop your tailbone under. On the inhale, lift your hips up high, coming onto your shoulders. Walk your shoulder blades in toward each other underneath your torso, clasp your hands together, and interlace your fingers. Press down through your feet and upper arms. Keep your knees hip-width apart and spin your inner thighs down toward the floor. It's very important not to let your knees splay out to the sides. Keep them directly above your heels at all times. Draw your belly in.

Gaze down to the tip of your nose. On the in breath expand your rib cage. On the out breath, drive the feet and upper arms down and the hips up higher.

Alignment:
- Feet are hip-width apart and parallel (or slightly splayed out for more comfort in your knees).

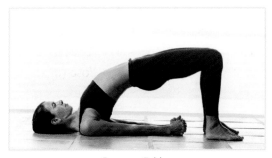

Pose 35: Bridge

- Stack your knees over your ankles.
- Contract your quadriceps, hamstrings, and buttocks.
- Spin your inner thighs down toward the floor.
- Root down through the soles of your feet and lift your hips high.
- Release your face and set your eyes to the tip of your nose.

Risk Factor: Letting the knees splay out or come forward past the toes puts strain on the knee ligaments.

Modification: If you cannot lift your hips up high, just do what you can. Work to your capacity, even if that means coming halfway up. If you feel strain in your knees, move your heels a little farther away from your sitting bones, or play with the splay of your feet.

Spiritual Focus: Have no agenda other than to be fully present. Use your breath to connect your mind to the here and now and watch the moments unfold. No matter how much stress, pressure, or adversity the moment at hand presents, stay in your body, stay with your breath. Every time your mind wanders, simply begin again. If you lose presence and launch into reactivity, it's OK; just notice it and begin again.

Connecting Vinyasa

After five breaths, release your hands and lower your hips to the mat. Relax for a few breaths, then repeat Bridge pose once more. Lower your hips again and stay as you are in preparation for the next pose, Wheel.

Pose 36: Wheel (Urdhva Dhanurasana)

Wheel is one of the most powerful poses in yoga practice. The entire front side of the body unfolds into a magnificent blossom. The muscles in the back of the legs and shoulders are especially strengthened and conditioned. This is one of the very best poses to open and release the tightness and tension in the upper back, chest, shoulders, and hip flexors. Your breathing apparatus is opened, which greatly increases the oxygen flow to your blood. You are also bringing love and life into your spine.

On a deeper level, Wheel inspires a sense of physical freedom, youthfulness, lightness, and joy. It can create tremendous emotional release.

Building Blocks: Lie on your back with your feet flat on the floor hip-width apart (same preparation as for Bridge pose). Place your

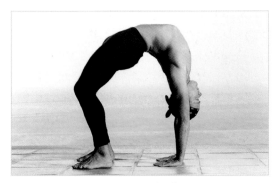
Pose 36: Wheel

hands flat next to your ears with the palms down and your fingertips toward your shoulders. Pull your elbows in so they are in line with your shoulder joints, then drop your shoulders down toward your buttocks.

Step one: Exhale and scoop your tail. On the inhalation, pressing down gently through the soles of your feet and hands, come onto the crown of your head at the floor. It is important to put your body weight into your hands and arms rather than sitting in your neck. If this is as far as you can comfortably go, that's fine; just hold here for five breaths. Straightening your arms may be difficult if your shoulders are tight, but they will stretch and open over time with practice.

Step two: Pull your elbows in so they are in line with your shoulder joints, then drop your shoulder blades down your back. It's very important that you find that movement before lifting up. Exhale here. Then, pressing down through the soles of your feet and your palms, inhale as you straighten your arms and launch up into a beautiful back-bend. Your head is heavy, your neck is free. This should feel so good! Spin your inner thighs down toward the floor to keep rooted and stable. Keep your knees drawn in toward each other at hip width—don't let them splay out. Your feet are as parallel as possible, but a slight splay is OK.

Wheel can be very intense, and you might become fatigued before you get to five full breaths. But remember, right when you want to give up, right when you perceive failure, that is the moment you are about to cross into new territory. Change is uncomfortable. And when you feel as if you've got to quit, that's probably the point at which you're looking right into the possibility of changing at some level. That's the time to stay calm and breathe deep. If you can stay with it in those difficult moments, you will grab the brass ring of transformation.

After five breaths, tuck your chin and slowly lower yourself from the top of your spine down to the bottom, then your hips. **Do not** bring your knees into your chest! A lot of teachers will tell you to do this, but that movement shocks your sacrum. Just keep the soles of your feet on the mat and your hips down (or come into Supta Baddha Konasana, the next pose).

Repeat Wheel pose three to six times. Yes, three to six times! The good news about backbends is that each one gets easier. With each one, you peel away a little more resistance. The final one may feel the most daunting, but it is what makes the difference between walking away at the end of your yoga practice and flying!

Alignment:

- Stack your knees over your heels.
- Wrap your elbows in toward each other at shoulder width.
- Drop your shoulder blades way down your back before lifting up.
- Root your four limbs down as you press your hips up.
- Press your hamstrings and hips up to the sky.
- Rotate your inner thighs toward the floor.
- Shift more weight into your legs.
- Let your neck hang free.
- Own every bone in your whole body.
- Relax your face and focus the lens of your eyes on the wall behind you.

Risk Factor: If you don't drop your shoulders down your back before lifting up, you risk straining your shoulders. You may not notice it at first, but over time and with consistent repetition of unhealthy movement you can create wear and tear on your shoulder joints. Dropping your scapulae stabilizes the shoulders. Distribute your weight on all four limbs rather than jamming into your shoulders.

Modification: Stay on the crown of your head with your arms at right angles. If you cannot do this, stay in Bridge pose until you are ready to move into the new territory of Wheel. Experiment with splaying your feet (*not* your knees) out a bit if you feel strain in your knees.

Spiritual Focus: Some people plant seeds in the spring and lose patience if they don't see results immediately. If you've committed for a season, see it through. You don't have to stay forever, but at least wait to see what blooms. What you see may surprise you and keep you for another season.

Connecting Vinyasa

After the final Wheel, lower yourself to your mat. While lying on your back with your shoulders on the mat, take a gentle twist, bringing both knees to one side and then the other, taking five breaths on each side. Then come to center and into the next pose, Supta Baddha Konasana.

Pose 37: Supta Baddha Konasana

Supta Baddha Konasana is another pose we refer to only by its Sanskrit name. It is a wonderful neutralizing pose, especially after the intensity of backbends. It soothes the nervous system, allowing the body some deep rest. It releases the lower back and hips while stretching the inner thigh muscles. As you drop into the floor and surrender to this pose, all of your internal organs and body systems are rebalanced and revitalized. This pose invites deep, authentic rest—a rare gift in our pressure-filled world.

From the resting position after Wheel, while lying on your back, bend your knees and bring the soles of your feet together,

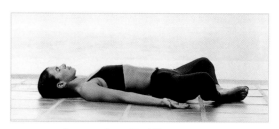
Pose 37: Supta Baddha Konasana

letting your legs and knees butterfly open to the sides. Your feet should be about one or two feet away from your groin. Scoop your tailbone under slightly, taking some of the arch out of your lower back. Let your belly drop. Lay your arms by your sides with your palms facing up (or, if you prefer, place your hands on your belly). Close your eyes, letting them relax in their sockets. Drop your mask, let go of your thoughts, relax deeply, and breathe.

Alignment:
- Drop your belly.
- Let the valley of your pelvis sink into the earth.
- Scoop your tailbone under, drawing the front of your pelvis up toward your ribs.
- Close your eyes.
- Let everything melt down.

Modification: If you feel strain in your knees, move your feet a little farther away from your groin. There is a natural arch in your back, but if it creates strain, place your feet flat on the floor.

Spiritual Focus: Fear knocked at the door, faith answered, and fear disappeared.

7. Abdominal Series: Stability

You are only as strong as your core. Strengthening your limbs will give you agility and stability in your movements, but building core muscles gives you a deeper seat of power. It is an inner strength that stabilizes every move you make. Abdominal work is key to any healthy yoga practice because strong abs take unnecessary pressure off your lower back. Your poses become much lighter and easier when you generate the effort from that strong core rather than from isolated muscles in your back and limbs. And the nice by-product is that you end up with really toned and sculpted abs!

The abdominal strengtheners we do here are yoga variations of fitness crunches. The difference between what we do and regular crunches is that power yoga abdominal work is global: It integrates and coordinates the upper, lower, and mid-body in such a way that it creates new patterns of stabilized movement that trains your body for motions like carrying groceries, picking up your kids, and reaching up into your closet. This real-life flexible strength allows you to walk through the world with grace and ease.

Pose 38: Scissor Legs and 60/30 Lift

This two-part pose tones and strengthens the entire abdominal wall.

Building Blocks: From the resting position, lie on your back, bring your knees into your chest and give them a squeeze. Cradle your head with your hands and extend your legs straight up to the sky. Lower your right leg down to one foot above the floor. Flex your feet and press through both of your legs. Lift your head and bring both shoulder blades off the floor. Inhale and get ready.

Exhale and contract your belly in toward the floor as you pulse your torso up for ten counts. As you lift up, contract your abdominal wall. Match your breath to your movements. Change legs and repeat on the left side for ten counts.

Next, bring both legs up and bring your arms out parallel to the floor (or you can keep cradling your head if your neck needs support), keeping your shoulder blades off the floor. Lower your legs down 30 degrees and hold for five breaths. Then lower your legs down another 30 degrees and again hold for five breaths. Then lower your legs until the heels are two inches off the floor and hold for the last five breaths. Rest in Supta Baddha Konasana.

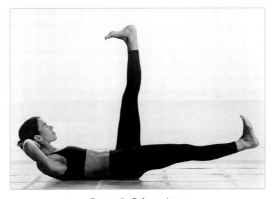

Pose 38: Scissor Legs

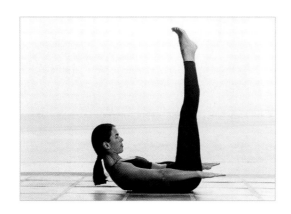

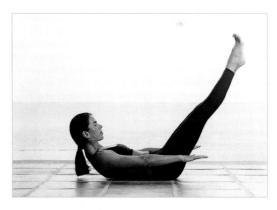

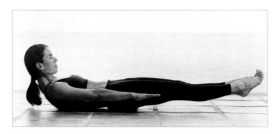

Pose 38: 60/30 Lift

Alignment:

- When holding your head, keep your forearms out to the side, not pulled in by your ears.
- Hold both shoulder blades off the floor for the entire sequence.
- Don't worry about flattening your back into the floor; the natural curvature of the spine is the healthiest position.

- Draw your belly to the floor.
- Keep your legs active.
- Press through the balls of your feet.

Risk Factor: Don't crank your neck; just let your head rest in your hands.

Modification: If you feel strain in the lower back, bend one knee and press the sole of that foot into the floor. Or experiment with bending both knees.

Spiritual Focus: In yoga, the body is considered a vehicle through which the world as a whole is transformed. A strong, healthy body is not meant to be a selfish end unto itself. To make our physical shape the end focus creates self-centeredness, disharmony, and disease. Rather, the body can be used as an instrument to express personal power for positive change in the world around us. That is the greatest inspiration we can have for building our core power.

Pose 39: Abdominal Twists

Abdominal Twists rewire the patterns of movement for graceful coordination and integrated force. They strengthen and tone the core muscles that are down deep as opposed to just the superficial ones—specifically the abdominal obliques, which are the support and stabilizing muscles for the lower back.

Building Blocks: After a few breaths in Supta Baddha Konasana, draw your knees up to your chest and give them a squeeze. If you

BARON BAPTISTE

want, you can rock back and forth a few times, forward and back, side to side, to massage your lower back. Then come onto your back with your knees in to your chest and lace your hands together under your head. Lift your shoulder blades off the floor, taking care not to strain your neck. Your head should be heavy, resting in your hands. Cradling your head, bring your elbows up to the outside of your knees.

On the out breath, straighten your right leg to a 45-degree angle and twist your right elbow to the outside of your left knee. Keep that lower shoulder blade raised, but don't crank your neck with your hands. Pull up with your abdominal muscles. Hold for three counts, then, on the in breath, come back to center, touching your elbows to the outside of your knees. Contract your belly and bring your hips and shoulders up when you draw in, as if you are closing an accordion.

Exhale your left leg out and spin your left elbow to the outside of your right knee. Hold, and on the inhale come back to center, elbows to the outside of your knees. On the exhale you extend and twist, on the inhale pull in and tuck up. Match breath to movement. The rhythm is: Inhale to center. Hold. Exhale, straighten and spin. Inhale to center. Hold. Exhale, straighten and spin. Be mindful, not mindless. Stay present to your breath and your body. The more difficult it is, the more you breathe!

Repeat for ten breaths, and on the last one, reach everything up—your legs, your

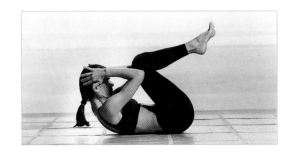

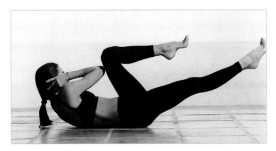

Pose 39: Abdominal Twist

hips, your head, your hands—everything up to the ceiling to the count of ten. Everything reaching except your belly, which contracts and presses back into the floor. Then relax your head, neck, and the soles of your feet back down to your mat and rest in Supta Baddha Konasana.

Risk Factor: Beware of wrenching your neck and overarching your lower back.

Modification: Raising your legs to a 60-degree angle during the twist will ease some of the intensity. You can also keep both knees bent throughout to whatever degree you need.

Spiritual Focus: In every moment, we are either finding ourselves or losing ourselves. We are either *now here* in our body, or *nowhere*. Connecting mind, movement, and breath will always lead you back to the now moment—the place where all true healing and growth is possible.

Pose 40: Boat Pose (Navasana)

This pose creates structural integration and balance while it strengthens and tones the abdominal wall and hip flexor muscles. It stabilizes the back and torso by strengthening the abdominal obliques bilaterally, which gives lower back support internally. In addition, it rinses the organs of the belly.

Building Blocks: Come to a sitting position. Contract your abdominal wall as you lift your legs and torso up, bringing your arms forward until they are parallel to the floor. The object is to balance on your tail and sitting bones, so you look like a "V." To help with balance, you can keep your hands on the floor until your legs and torso are balanced, then extend your arms. If you need to bend your knees a bit, you can do that. But the ideal is to have your legs straight.

The lift and balance in this pose comes from your abdomen, back, and hips. Really engage those muscles to stabilize and lift your torso and your legs. At the same time, draw your sternum up to the sky. Squeeze your legs, press your inner thighs together, and activate your feet. Focus your eyes on a point in front of you and sail your beautiful boat!

Hold Navasana for five breaths, then bend your knees, cross your feet in front of you, keeping them raised off the floor. Press your hands down on the floor next to your hips, contract your abs, and lift your whole body off the floor for one breath. Come down and repeat the sequence—Navasana and then the crossed ankle lift—for a total of three to five sets. At the end lie flat on your back with the soles of your feet together in Supta Baddha Konasana.

Alignment:
- Legs are straight and alive.
- Abdominal muscles are engaged.
- Lift your sternum toward the ceiling.
- Reach your arms forward. They should be parallel to the floor.
- Establish a calm, steady, powerful gaze.

Risk Factor: Beware of rounding or hyperextending (overarching) your lower back. Emphasize your abdominal lock and dropping the front ribs down.

Modification: Either bend your knees slightly, or work with one foot on the floor if lifting both legs feels too strenuous. Another option is to keep your hands at the floor as you extend your legs straight. For the cross and lift, place one block on each side of your body to give some extra height.

Spiritual Focus: Your breath is what anchors you. It is always right there under your nose. Watch its ebb and flow as you glide through the crystal-clear waters of your equanimous mind.

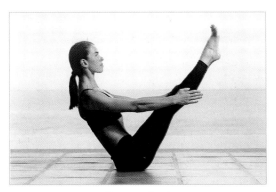

Pose 40: Boat

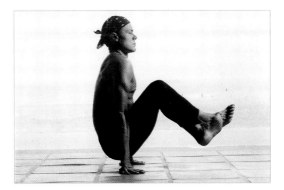

Boat, crossed ankle lift

8. Inversion Series: Rejuvenation

Any pose where you bring your head below your heart is considered an inversion. Inversions are a very important part of yoga practice. They flush the organs in the head and upper torso with fresh, oxygenated blood. They activate and electrify the glands that govern the immune system and the internal pharmacy, creating vitality and vigor. They drain the fluid from the legs and hips to create suppleness in the lower body. Over a period of years, whether you are inactive, athletic, or do a strong yoga practice, if you are not turning your world upside down with inversions, you tend to dry out. Your body will get stiffer and you will lose agility and mobility in your everyday movements. Inversions keep your body supple and elastic.

Reversing the flow of gravity moves lymph—the body's "sewage"—through your system so metabolic waste can be released. It activates the thyroid and parathyroid glands, which boost and balance your metabolism.

There are many different inversion poses, including headstand, forearm balance, and handstands, and as you progress and mature in your practice I suggest you research and practice these more advanced inversions. But for the sake of creating a safe practice for you at home, I've chosen the three that are relatively simply but powerfully effective: Shoulder Stand, Plow, and Deaf Man's Pose.

Pose 41: Shoulder Stand (Sarvangasana)

The Shoulder Stand drains the legs of metabolic waste and allows fresh, oxygen-rich blood to circulate through the head, heart, and chest. It clears and stimulates the sinuses, thyroid, and parathyroid glands. It infuses the whole body with radiance and makes you feel bright yet serene.

Building Blocks: Lying on your back, bring your knees into your chest. Contract your abdominal muscles and, on an exhalation, bring your legs and hips up high to the sky, rolling onto the back of your shoulders. Bring your hands to your lower back and

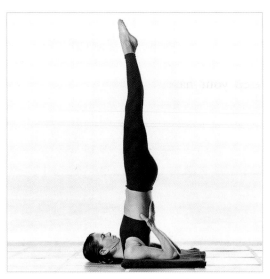

Pose 41: Shoulder Stand

- Press your shoulders down into your mat.
- Walk your elbows and shoulder blades in toward each other.
- Use your hands to support your lower back.
- Lift the weight of your body upward and away from your shoulders, head, and neck.
- Move your tailbone into your body and up toward the ceiling.
- Spiral your inner thighs toward the wall in front of you.
- Contract your abdominal muscles.
- Open your chest.
- Relax your neck and throat.
- Lift into your heels.
- Let your face relax.
- Soften and set your eyes at the tip of your nose or on your toes.

walk your elbows and shoulder blades in toward each other. Press up through the soles of your feet, using your hands to support your hips and lift them higher.

Ideally, you want your body to be in a straight vertical line. Use your abdominal muscles to pull your legs, hips, and pubic bone high, and drive down through your elbows. Rotate your thighs in and toward the wall in front of you. Keep your ankle bones touching and your feet alive. Look straight up, **never to the right or left.**

A nice way to work this pose for greater support is to place a folded blanket under your shoulders only, with your head on the floor. Never place a blanket, towel, or any other object under your neck in an inversion! Make sure the blanket is folded evenly.

Stay in Shoulder Stand for ten breaths. From here, you will move directly into the next pose, Plow.

Risk factor: **Do not turn your head once you are in this pose!** Keep your chin in line with your spine and look straight up to avoid injuring your neck. You can also put too much strain on your neck by not drawing your weight upward.

Modification: If you have a weak lower back or neck problems or feel any strain in your neck, I encourage you to take this modification, which provides many of the same benefits. Lie on your back, arms to your sides, and simply lift your legs straight in the air to a perpendicular line. Keep your hips on the mat and hold here for the full five breaths. As with the regular Shoulder

Stand, rotate your inner thighs in and engage a strong abdominal core.

Spiritual Focus: Forget what the pose looks like. The question is: What does it feel like? Your goal should be the opposite of glory-bound poses and performance. It is only when you shrink from all image-building processes that you begin to discover the prize of inner peace and authentic personal power.

Pose 42: Plow (Halasana)

Plow is an incredible stretch for the entire back, from the sacrum all the way up to the shoulders. It soothes, calms, and nurtures the vital internal body parts and nervous system.

Building Blocks: From Shoulder Stand, use your core power to slowly lower your straight legs to the floor behind your head. They may not reach the floor, and that's fine; just go as far as you can and hold there. That is your edge in this pose. Remember, the thing that blocks your path *is* your path! If your feet touch the floor, bring your arms toward the front

wall, interlacing your fingers and squeezing your elbows to a straight position. If your feet cannot reach the floor, just keep your hands at your lower back for support.

Relax your face and gaze forward to your navel. Breathe deep and free for five breaths.

Alignment:
- Walk your shoulder blades in toward each other.
- Press your pubic bone upward.
- Press your quadriceps up toward the ceiling.
- Spin your inner thighs up to the ceiling.
- Set your eyes gently on your navel.

Risk Factor: As in Shoulder Stand, it is very important that you do not turn your head to either side while in this pose, or you will wrench your neck.

Modification: You can set a folded blanket evenly beneath your shoulders for more support, or lower down with bent knees if you feel strain in your lower back. If you get stuck on your way back and your feet do not reach the mat, you can either set your feet on a wall behind you or just stay at that point and hold.

Spiritual Focus: Your meditative journey will be in two directions at once—inward and outward. To the degree that you come out of your head and are present in your body, you will see what to aim for in the tangible

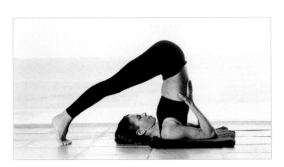

Pose 42: Plow

world. You will see what direction to take, how far to go, when to push and when to surrender. As you journey inward, you reflect your light outward.

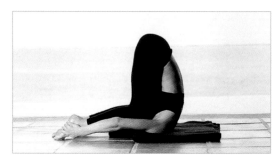
Pose 43: Deaf Man's Pose

Pose 43: Deaf Man's Pose (Karnapidasana)

In this pose you restore the wisdom of the body and create sanctuary, deep release, and biochemical balance. The spine will surrender into this profound space-enhancing stretch.

Building Blocks: From Plow, bend and drop your knees in toward your ears. Sweep your arms out and around and take hold of your feet. You can experiment with bringing your hands to your heels, ankles, calves, or to the base of your back to make this comfortable. Your toes can be pointed or turned under. Relax into this shape and breathe deep and smooth.

Stay here for ten to twenty breaths, gradually increasing the amount of time you spend in this pose. Eventually you want to hold this pose for a full minute.

Alignment:
- Hold your feet, ankles, or calves.
- Come onto your shoulders.
- Draw your knees in toward your ears.

Risk Factor: Neck weaknesses need to be carefully observed here. Dilute the pressure as needed, or skip this pose entirely.

Modification: Place a blanket beneath your shoulders with your head remaining directly on the floor. Bring your knees to your forehead and your heels up toward your hips instead of bringing them to the floor.

Spiritual Focus: Seal off the distractions around you and listen to the sound of your breath. Nothing to hear but the beautiful rhythm of your inhalations and exhalations. Follow its thread into the deepest place of restoration within you.

Connecting Vinyasa

Slowly and gently roll out of this pose onto your back, bringing your hands to your knees. Gently roll up and back five times. On the fifth time, bring your hands to the floor in front of you and with great momentum walk or jump your feet back to Low Push-Up (9) position. Inhale to Upward Facing Dog (10) and exhale to Downward Facing Dog (2). You are now in position for the next pose, Half Pigeon.

9. Hip Series: Opening

In the hip-opening series we focus on releasing and unlocking the adductor and rotator muscles of the buttocks. In addition, hip-opening poses dissolve lower back tension, knee discomfort, sciatic nerve pain, and improve blood flow to the lumbar spine, intestines, and reproductive glands. They create greater overall agility and freedom of movement.

The hips are the emotional storage depot for the body. They house a good portion of your tension and stress, and as you start releasing your pelvis and softening that tissue, the rest of your body effortlessly shifts into a natural order of alignment. Sometimes just by releasing tension and tightness we create healing and balance, working out the chinks and kinks in our bodies. If you have a neck problem, knee problem, low-back problem, headaches, or whatever, it's amazing how all those aches, pains, and misalignments can disappear once you open up the hips.

When I worked with professional football players, who were very muscular and tight (most couldn't touch their toes), I immediately started them on hip-opening poses. After only a few sessions, they started to loosen up and had more mobility in their entire bodies than they had had in years! I like to call the hips the "mother of all movement," for obvious reasons.

Hip openers will bring resistance up faster than almost any other series of poses. They are very much in your face as far as the pain, but if you sit with the pain and don't fight it, it passes. It passes through and out of you forever. Remember, the yogic principle that nothing is per-

manent. If you just breathe through these pains of purification, you will venture into whole new territories of growth. You reach down into the hidden pockets of tissue, to the places where your deepest power lies waiting to be tapped. Lifelong barriers melt away as the tissue releases and you gently peel away layers of old, useless bundles of energy and information.

I teach three hip openers in power yoga: Half-Pigeon, Double Pigeon, and Frog.

Pose 44: Half Pigeon
(Adho Mukha Eda Pada Rajakapotasana)

Half Pigeon releases the periformis muscle, which is notorious for getting very tight in athletes and runners. If you are a professional "sitter," this pose will also help keep those muscles from getting brittle, stiff, and sore.

Building Blocks: From Downward Facing Dog, look up between your hands and step your right foot to the outside of your left hand. Then drop your right knee near the right hand and drop your right hip down to the floor. You want to get your shin as parallel to the front edge of your mat as possible. Depending on the tightness in your hips, this can be difficult, so work to your degree of comfort. Flex your right foot. If you like, you can place your left palm on the sole of your right foot. Last, relax your upper body forward over your right shin, bringing your arms out straight in front of you and your forehead to the mat if it will reach. Work on squaring the

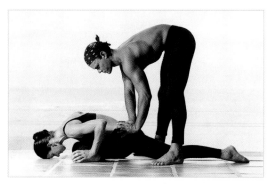

Pose 44: Half Pigeon (assisted)

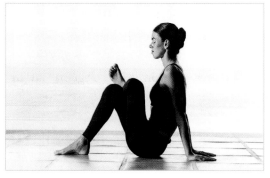

Pigeon, modification

front side of your torso down toward the floor. Your back leg and foot should be stretched straight back.

You want to maintain as much of a center line as possible through your hips, so roll your left hip down toward the mat.

Channel your breath down into your hips and buttock, softening and releasing the tissue. This should feel so deep . . . so good . . . so freeing! If you feel fidgety or uncomfortable, it's just anxiety coming up. But if you can recognize it as such and breathe through it, the discomfort will dissolve like snow in the summer sun. Tune in, breathe, relax. Break up tension, break with the old and break through to the new!

Alignment:

- Front leg is at a 90-degree angle (or less, depending on the flexibility of your hips or if it bothers the knee).
- Back leg extends straight behind you.
- Press the tops of all five toes on the back foot into the floor.
- Flex your front foot.
- Press the upper hip down.

- Rotate your back inner thigh upward.
- Bring your forehead to the mat if it reaches.
- Soften your eyes and gaze down.

Spiritual Focus: Slam on your mental brakes and expand into full acceptance of the present moment—everything you are feeling and what is happening. Don't try to change anything. Just breathe, witness, and let go. Allow this moment to be exactly as it is, and watch with a quiet mind as each new moment unfolds. Allow yourself to be exactly as you are, so that you may break through your resistance.

Connecting Vinyasa

Breathe for five breaths, then bring your upper body back up slowly, resting on your hands. Leave your legs as they are in preparation for the next pose, Double Pigeon.

Pose 45: Double Pigeon
(Dwapada Rajakapotasana)

Double Pigeon is a deep hip stretch that opens you up. Sometimes it is difficult to get into this pose. Take the time you need, because the rewards are large.

Building Blocks: From Half Pigeon, sit up and slowly bring the back leg up and around, stacking your left shin directly on top of your right shin. Ideally you want to get the upper foot to the outside of the opposite thigh so it is hanging in the air, not resting on top of your leg. Flex both feet. Walk your hands forward and relax down, letting your head hang forward, or set both hands on the upper knee and lean into it. If you can, bring your forehead down to your mat. Now just breathe way down deep into your pelvis as though it were hollow. Let the beautiful cleansing wind sweep away any tension that you are holding there.

Alignment:

- Stack your shins on top of each other, legs at right angles.
- Bring the anklebone of the top foot to the outside of the lower thigh.
- Flex your feet.
- Lengthen your spine.
- Drop your mask and soften your eyes.

Risk Factor: Pointing or collapsing your feet strains your knees and/or ankles. Keep your feet firmly flexed, lengthening through the heels.

Modification: If this pose is difficult for you, try this variation: From a seated position, set your feet flat on the floor with your

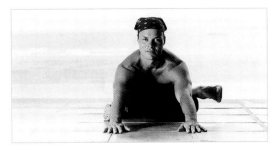

Pose 45: Double Pigeon

knees bent. Bring one foot up to the opposite thigh. Set your hands on the floor behind your hips and walk them in, moving your torso toward your legs until you feel a deep stretch in your butt cheek.

Spiritual Focus: Thoreau said, "Direct your eyes inward and you'll find a thousand regions in your mind yet undiscovered. Travel them and be an expert in home cosmography." Where are the uncharted regions within you?

Connecting Vinyasa

After five breaths, sweep the top leg back into Half Pigeon again. Set your palms on the floor and step back to Downward Facing Dog. Then bring your left foot forward to the outside of your right hand and repeat Half Pigeon and Double Pigeon on this side. When you are done, release your legs and come to a seated position for the next position, Frog.

Pose 46: Frog Pose (Bhekasana)

Frog pose reaches into and releases the muscles and tissue deep within the hips and groin. This pose is an intense, rejuvenating stretch that can be emotionally charged. After a long hold, your whole body will feel invigorated and infused with light.

Building Blocks: Face the side wall. Double up your mat on each end and stand on your knees with your shins pressing into the floor. Place your knees as far apart as you can, as if you're doing a straddle-split on your knees. Go out to your maximum edge. Turn your heels out so the inner edges of your feet are against the mat and flex your feet. Your thighs and shins should form right angles. Check to make sure your heels are in line with your knees.

Come down on your forearms. Move your hips back toward the wall behind you until you feel a good stretch. Your head is heavy, your breathing deep. Really go to the potent point of stretch and stress and breathe that purifying wind down into the cavern of your body. You're here for a little while, so just relax with it. Don't fight, don't panic. You're perfectly safe in this pose. This is a wonderful opportunity to create a structural and emotional shift. It will change your body, but the willingness to hang in there is what will rewire your mind and ultimately change your life.

Hold this pose for twenty-five deep and powerful life-changing breaths.

Alignment:
- Keep your heels in line with your knees and your legs at right angles.
- Scoop your tailbone down and under.

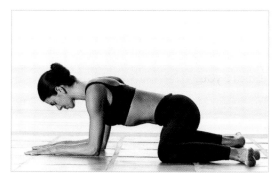

Pose 46: Frog

- Gently contract your belly upward.
- Press your hips backward with every breath you take.
- Let your head drop.
- Melt your mask.
- Close your eyes or soften them to a spot between your forearms.

Risk Factor: Do not collapse into your lower back; stay lifted at your belly. There should be zero pain in the knee joints. If necessary, put more padding beneath your knees.

Modification: If your hips are really tight, you can roll up a blanket or use a bolster under your chest and belly. Eventually your hips will open as you continue to practice, so with time you won't need the bolster.

Spiritual Focus: If you are not willing, you cannot open. Focus on healing and let the rest go. Notice how old patterns of attack and reactivity come up and just let them go. If you want your body to relax, it's simple: Just relax your mind. If you want to let go of the baggage you are holding in your body, let go of the baggage in your mind. Be willing and all possibility unfolds before you.

Connecting Vinyasa

Come out of this pose by simply lying forward on your belly for a beautiful release from the deep hip work. Take a few breaths and then lie on your back, pulling your knees into your chest. Then come up into a seated position, scoot back to the middle of the mat, and extend your legs out in front of you. You are now in position for the Forward Bending Series.

10. Forward Bending Series: Release

Forward bends bring new energy and tone into the vital organs of the body. They lengthen and create a natural traction through the back side of the torso and dissolve tightness in the hamstrings, buttocks, and lower back. These cooling poses slow the pulse and unclutter the brain. Since they can be held for long periods, you have the time to really feel and relax deeply into your body.

There are two forward bending poses: Seated Single Leg Extension and Seated Forward Bend. Then you'll take Tabletop and Fish Pose as neutralizing poses.

Pose 47: Seated Single Leg Extension (Janu Sirsasana)

This pose releases the calves, hamstrings, glutes, and back and improves blood circulation in the legs. It dissolves restlessness and irritability and soothes the brain and nervous system.

Building Blocks: From the upright seated position, bring your left heel in to the inside of your right thigh. Keep your right foot active and press the top of your right thigh into the floor. On the exhalation, reach forward and grab your foot with both hands if you can (if not, grab your ankle). Breathe in and lift halfway up to a straight back, then exhale and reach forward as you bend down.

You may want to try a little extra twisting action in this pose, so work your left ear down toward your right knee as you lift your right ribs up high. You may even want to bring your right hand to the floor to the outside of your hip to leverage your twist. Breathe deeply for five breaths, lift back up, and do the same steps on the other side for another five breaths.

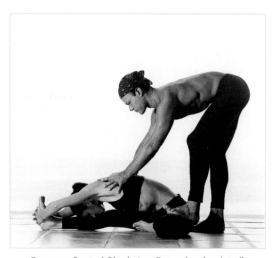

Pose 47: Seated Single Leg Extension (assisted)

Alignment:

- Keep the foot of your extended leg active.
- Press the top of the thigh of the extended leg into the floor.
- Hinge at your hips.
- Pull your belly in and up.
- Relax your neck, face, and eyes.

Risk Factor: Bending at the waist can strain the lower spine. Hinge at the hips.

Modification: If you are really tight, bend the knee of your extended leg.

Spiritual Focus: Making an internal shift is like dropping a pebble in a pond. Every microshift ripples into and through your mind, your body, and your life, growing ever bigger and more powerful.

Connecting Vinyasa

After five breaths on the left side, come up and extend both legs out for the next pose, the Seated Forward Bend.

Pose 48: Seated Forward Bend (Paschimottanasana)

This is a wonderful countermovement to everything you have done up until now. It lengthens and releases the back side of the body and leaves you feeling neutral, balanced, and restored.

Building Blocks: Sitting upright with both legs extended out in front of you, reach under your butt and pull your sitting muscles out laterally so you come right onto your sitting bones. Your legs are together, ankles touching. Press the tops of your thighs down toward the floor and flex your feet. On the exhalation, reach forward, hinging from the hips, and grab your feet, ankles, or legs with both hands. (If you can't grab your feet, try bending your knees, holding your feet, and then gradually pressing the tops of your thighs down to the floor to an intense yet comfortable degree.) Inhale and lift halfway up to a straight back, then exhale and fold forward. Keep your feet active and toes fanned. Let your elbows bend out to the side.

On the inhalation, use your hands to pull you forward, lengthening through the spine. On the exhalation, bring your torso down toward your knees. Inhale reach, exhale torso down. Don't worry if your spine is rounded. Just try to lengthen it gradually and smoothly over time. Drop your head and release your neck. Soften your eyes and set your gaze between your legs.

It's important that you focus on bending from the hips, not the waist. Pulling from your waist puts unnecessary strain on the lower back. It's not about how far you go into this pose, but rather how you hold it in general: the compassion, intention, and overall integration of your movement. Hold this pose for ten breaths, coming back up to a seated position on an inhalation.

Alignment:

- Activate your feet and press through the mounds of the big toes.

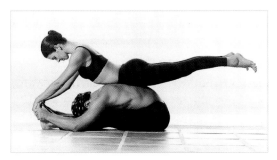

Pose 48: Seated Forward Bend (assisted)

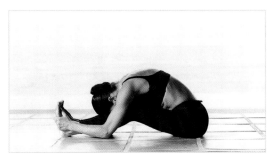

Seated Forward Bend, modification

- Press the tops of your thighs toward the floor.
- Spin your inner thighs downward.
- Hinge at your hips.
- Pull your chest away from your hips.
- Relax your shoulders.
- Neck is neutral and free.
- Gaze to your legs.

Risk Factor: Bending at the waist can strain the spine. Work at hinging from your hips and extending through your spine.

Modification: Bend your knees. Or you can use a towel or strap around your feet as an extended handle.

Spiritual Focus: Some poses may lead you to think that yoga practice is too simple to deliver the results we need. But after a while you realize that we are much more likely to succeed *because* the program is simple and straightforward. We come to understand that it is far better to work at our own level of ability and do a fixed set of basic poses in a consistent and healthy way than to try many different things and fail.

Yoga practice reminds us of the value and power of simplicity in personal growth.

Pose 49: Tabletop (Purvottanasana)

Tabletop neutralizes forward bends by releasing the back and opening up the front of the torso. It also stretches and tones the muscles in the front of the shoulders and biceps. This pose creates an overall feeling of release and expansion.

Building Blocks: From a seated position with your legs straight out in front of you, bring your hands back about twelve inches behind your hips, shoulder-width apart. Place your palms flat with your fingers facing forward. On the inhalation, press down through your arms and hands, straightening your elbows and lifting your hips up. Press all ten toes into the floor and lift your hips high. Drop your head back so the crown of your head is facing the floor. Gaze to the back wall and breathe deep and free.

Alignment:
- Press your palms flat.
- Straighten your arms and stack your shoulders over your wrists.

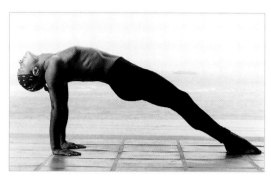

Pose 49: Tabletop

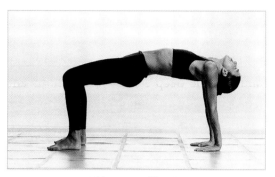

Tabletop, modification

- Move your shoulder blades in toward each other.
- Press all ten toes into the floor.
- Enthusiasm through your thighs!
- Gaze softly to the wall behind you with a timeless awareness.

Modification: If it is difficult to lift your hips upward, bend your knees and walk your heels in under your knees. In this variation, you want your body from your chest to your knees to be parallel to the floor, like a table. If it hurts your neck to drop your head back, simply bring your chin up toward your chest.

Spiritual Focus: Step back from judgment and you will marvel at what transpires through you. If you are open, you will find more faith in what you do not know than in what you do know.

Connecting Vinyasa

On the fifth exhalation, lower your hips back down to a seated position in preparation for Fish pose.

Pose 50: Fish Pose (Matsyasana)

Fish pose is a wonderful and powerful counterbalancing pose that releases the muscles in the back and reopens the throat, chest, and entire front side of the torso, bringing the body back into balance. This pose also helps to redirect the blood flow through the thyroid and parathyroid glands.

Building Blocks: From a seated position, place your hands under your sitting muscles, palms facing down. Lean back until your forearms are down on the floor. Walk your elbows and forearms in toward each other, shimmy your shoulder blades in toward each other. On the inhale, raise your heart muscle high and arch your back, lower your head back and slide back until the crown is resting on the floor. Create a big, beautiful bend in your upper back, opening your throat and heart to the heavens. Root your shoulders down and away from your ears and lift through your chest. (As in Camel, your shoulder blades are like giant hands pressing your chest upward.)

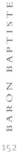

Point your toes and activate your thighs. This stretch should feel so good!

Gaze to a point on the wall behind you and breathe deep for five inhalations and exhalations. Fill your lungs completely with sweet oxygen so your entire being is full of breath, full of life. After the fifth exhalation, inhale, lift your head up, tuck your chin, slowly release your arms, and lower back down to a horizontal resting position.

Alignment:
- Point and activate your toes.
- Keep your feet together, inner anklebones touching.
- Root your forearms and shoulders down into the floor.
- Engage your thighs.
- Root the hips down and lift your heart muscle high.
- Gaze with soothing and steady focus to a point behind you.

Modification: If you have pain or strain in your neck, try working with your head off the floor, chin at your chest.

Spiritual Focus: Speaking from your heart comes from a single-minded attention to your intuition in the moment. From this inner space springs forth a steady flow of honesty and insight. When we are upset, we lose our focus, and our speech no longer flows gracefully from the ground of our being.

Fish pose stimulates and opens the

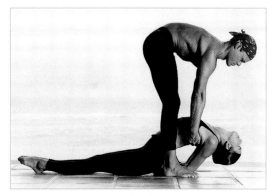

Pose 50: Fish (assisted)

throat and heart area—the energy center of self-expression and intuition. Inspiration may burst forth, or you may suddenly become aware of truths you have not been speaking, either to yourself or others. Give conscious attention to whatever arises.

Connecting Vinyasa

Release your arms and lie on your back with your arms resting by your sides. You are now ready for the final part of the practice, Surrender to Gravity.

11. Surrender to Gravity Series: Deep Rest

The Surrender to Gravity Series is the closing sequence of the practice. You've made it! You have done your part in this practice; now it's just time to let go and let the universe meet you halfway. You've allowed a lot to happen just by opening up honestly, by challenging yourself to be more, by breathing deeply, by letting go of all the games and headstuff you originally brought with you to the mat. You've crossed the rivers of resistance in your mind, challenged yourself to climb emotional and spiritual mountains. And now, as Goethe promised centuries ago, "Over all the mountain tops is peace."

There are three poses in the Surrender to Gravity sequence: Dead Bug pose, Supine Twist, and the final resting pose, Savasana.

Pose 51: Dead Bug Pose
(Urdhva Mukha Upavista Konasana)

Dead Bug pose gives a final stretch to the hips, hamstrings, and inner thighs, and also releases the lower spine. It slows the heart rate and brings the body to a restorative and resting state. You are completely supported here by gravity.

Building Blocks: From a horizontal prone position, inhale and bring your knees up to your chest. Grab the inner edges of your feet, thumbs facing down toward your heels. Very gently pull your feet, knees, and quadriceps toward the floor. Your ankles should be stacked directly over your

knees. Roll your tailbone down toward your mat and lengthen your spine into the floor. You should feel a release in your spine and a good stretch in your hips, inner thighs, and hamstrings.

Allow your belly to drop. Now just relax into infinite awareness and breathe. Be really still . . . be really dead! Be the poster child for Raid! After five breaths, hug your knees back into your chest and stay here in preparation for the next pose, Supine Twist.

Alignment:
- Stack your ankles over your knees.
- Spread your thighs to the outer edges of your torso.
- Pull the soles of your feet downward.
- Move your tailbone down toward the floor.
- Lengthen the line of your spine flat into the floor.
- Soften your belly.
- Bring your chin toward your chest, lengthening your neck.
- Soften or close your eyes and melt into the brightness of your mind.

Spiritual Focus: You can't grab the next trapeze until you release the present one. Just let go!

Pose 52: Supine Twist

This final twist rinses away any remaining tension. It integrates everything you've done by balancing and releasing on every level. It flushes the middle of the body and

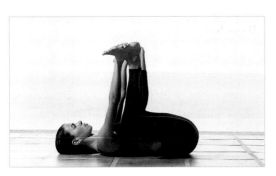

Pose 51: Dead Bug

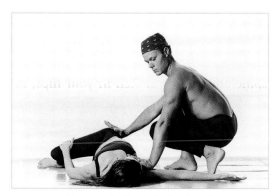
Pose 52: Supine Twist (assisted)

spine with nutrient-rich blood and helps to soothe a restless and emotional mind, inviting a new sense of serenity and peace.

Building Blocks: Straighten your left leg on the floor and pull your right knee into your chest. Exhale and spin your right knee over to the outer left side of your body. Open your right arm out like a wing and look over your right shoulder. Close your eyes and just rest. There is nothing else to do now but surrender.

Breathe deeply into the lower abdominal and pelvic cavities. Breathe into the lower back and kidney area. Ring out your spine and vital organs like a sponge. This is your time to cleanse and release. On the inhalation, breathe in that crystal-clear, purifying wind. On the exhalation, breathe away all the toxins and impurities.

After five breaths, bring your right leg back to center on the next inhalation. Reverse your legs and take another five breaths with your right leg extended. Return to center, hug both knees into your chest—go ahead, give them a good

squeeze—and then release them both down to the floor. Relax like never before.

Alignment:
- Create one long, straight line from the crown of your head to the sole of your extended foot.
- Twist until it feels good.
- Try to keep both shoulders on the floor.
- Close your eyes.

Risk Factor: Don't force the twist and strain your back; be gentle.

Modification: If this twist is too intense for your middle or lower back, move your bent knee down lower, toward the extended foot. Or if you need to, bend both knees and twist to the side with them pressed together. This will dilute the intensity of the movement.

Spiritual Focus: We tend to think that surrender is giving up our power. But surrender is anything but passive. It isn't throwing away our power. It's expanding it through faith and a willingness to let go of all we think we know . . . all we struggle to do . . . all we believe we need to accomplish.

Pose 53: Savasana

Savasana, which we refer to by its Sanskrit name only, signals the end of the asana practice and the gateway to a deeper, meditative state—a new beginning. Deeper rest shifts the brainwaves into the alpha state—

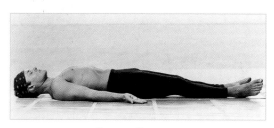
Pose 53: Savasana

the state of creativity, spiritual awakening, and peak performance. Even the smallest taste of this sensation rewires us toward a healthier and more powerful mode of being.

Building Blocks: Lie on your back with your legs straight and separated about twelve inches apart. Let your feet relax and splay out. Place your arms alongside your body, about six inches away from you, palms facing up. Roll your shoulder blades in toward each other—this allows your chest to expand and your breathing to shift profoundly. Pull your head out of your neck, your arms away from your shoulders, and your legs away from your hips. Lengthen your spine into the floor but allow the curvatures to take their natural form. Really feel the floor beneath you and your contact with it. Make whatever adjustments you need to feel comfortable here and let go. With every breath let your body fall deeper into the floor.

You've done your part. You've met the universe halfway. Now let every fiber of every muscle relax and release, and let magic happen. Close your eyes and just be still. Let go of your thoughts. It's just you and your breath now. Nowhere to go. Nowhere else to be but here now, in this moment. Nothing left to do but surrender. Just bask in your healing yogic glow and know that there is nothing more important than this moment and your own authentic, radiant being.

Stay here for as long as you like. Ideally ten to twenty minutes, to let your nervous system assimilate all the good you have done in your practice.

Alignment:
- Drop your brain.
- Close your eyes.
- Drop your belly.
- Release your whole body.
- Open your ears and really hear.
- Be in the now.

Modification: If your lower back aches, set your feet flat on the floor and/or prop up your torso with blankets. You can also place a rolled-up blanket under your knees.

Spiritual Focus: When you fully embrace this moment as an opportunity to heal, you tap into an energy that pushes you forward in physical endeavors. Our ultimate achievement comes not from what we do, what we accomplish, or what we accumulate, but rather from who we are—and that can change simply by having an internal shift. True success is not about anything more than truly living a life that works on all levels, not just for us, but for the world.

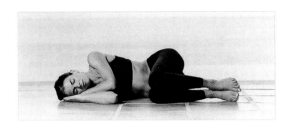

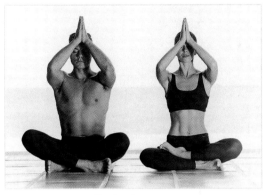

Closing Sequence

To Close Your Practice

Keep your eyes closed throughout this movement. When you are ready, roll onto your right side from Savasana into a fetal position with your knees to your chest. Stay here for as long as it feels right, then very slowly come up to a seated, cross-legged position. Bring your hands together in a prayerlike position at your heart center for a minute of stillness. If you'd like, you can chant "om" three times deeply as a way to create a peaceful harmony in your breathing and hormonal systems.

Then slowly bring your hands up to your third-eye center at your forehead. Breathe and invite in the light. We end all our practices by quietly saying "namaste," an acknowledgment of the light in ourselves and in all those around us.

Overview of the Poses

Integration Series
Child's Pose
Ragdoll
Downward Facing Dog

Sun Salutation A
Samasthiti
Mountain Pose
Standing Forward Bend
Halfway Lift
High Push-Up
Low Push-Up
Upward Facing Dog
Downward Facing Dog
Jump Forward
Halfway Lift
Standing Forward Bend
Mountain Pose
Samasthiti

Sun Salutation B
Samasthiti
Thunderbolt
Standing Forward Bend
Halfway Lift
High Push-Up
Low Push-Up
Upward Facing Dog
Downward Facing Dog
Warrior I, right leg forward.
High to Low Push-Up, Upward Facing Dog to
    Downward Facing Dog
Warrior I, left leg forward
High to Low Push-Up, Upward Facing Dog to
    Downward Facing Dog

Jump Forward
Thunderbolt

On the third round of Sun Salutation B, add Warrior II after Warrior I and end the vinyasa in Samastithi.

Warrior Series
Crescent Lunge
Revolving Crescent Lunge
Extended Side Angle
Side Plank
Prayer Twist
Gorilla Pose
Crow Pose

Balancing Series
Eagle Pose
Standing Leg Raise, Front
Standing Leg Raise, Side
Airplane Pose
Dancer's Pose
Tree Pose

Triangle Series
Triangle Pose
Twisting Triangle
Reverse Namaste Forward Bend
Standing Straddle Bend

Backbending Series
Locust
Bow
Camel
Bridge
Wheel
Supta Baddha Konasana

Abdominal Series
Scissor Legs and 60/30 Lift
Abdominal Twists
Boat Pose

Inversions
Shoulder Stand
Plow
Deaf Man's Pose

Hip Series
Half Pigeon
Double Pigeon
Frog

Forward Bends
Single Seated Leg Extention
Seated Leg Extension
Tabletop
Fish Pose

Surrender to Gravity
Dead Bug Pose
Supine Twist
Savasana

How to Design a Practice to Fit Your Schedule

I recognize that not everyone has ninety minutes every day to practice yoga, and that some days you will need to tailor your practice to fit into your schedule. Here is the formula to use when creating your modified practice.

1. Start with the Integration Series.
2. Do two Sun Salutation A.

3. Do one Sun Salutation B.
4. Choose one or more of the eleven posture series (Integration, Warrior, Inversions, Hip Openers, etc.) and do all the poses in that series. However, if you do more than one series, be sure to do them in the order in which they are arranged in the book. For example, if you choose to do the Backbending Series and the Hip Openers, do the Backbending Series first. If you choose to do Forward Bends and the Triangle Series, do the Triangle Series first.
5. End with at least five minutes in Savasana.

You can choose which series to do based on how your energy feels, or on what you physically or emotionally feel you need that day, or a combination of the two. For example:

- If you are tired or in need of an energy boost, do the Warrior series.
- If you are wired and want to wind down, do the Surrender to Gravity series.

- If your back feels stiff, do the Backbending series. Backbends are also particularly good to do if you feel emotionally constricted or burdened, as they open the chest area.
- If you have been sitting at your desk for a long stretch of time and feel cramped, you can do the Hip Opener series.

One note of caution: If you can only do modified practices, try to vary the series you do from day to day. You don't want to concentrate on only one part of the body. Yoga is a global exercise that is meant to work the entire body, and overdeveloping one area is no better than ignoring another entirely.

Don't skip your practice altogether just because you don't have time to do a full ninety minutes, or try to do more than ninety minutes when you have the time. Remember, it's better to do a little bit of yoga often if you are unable to do a full, well-rounded practice consistently.

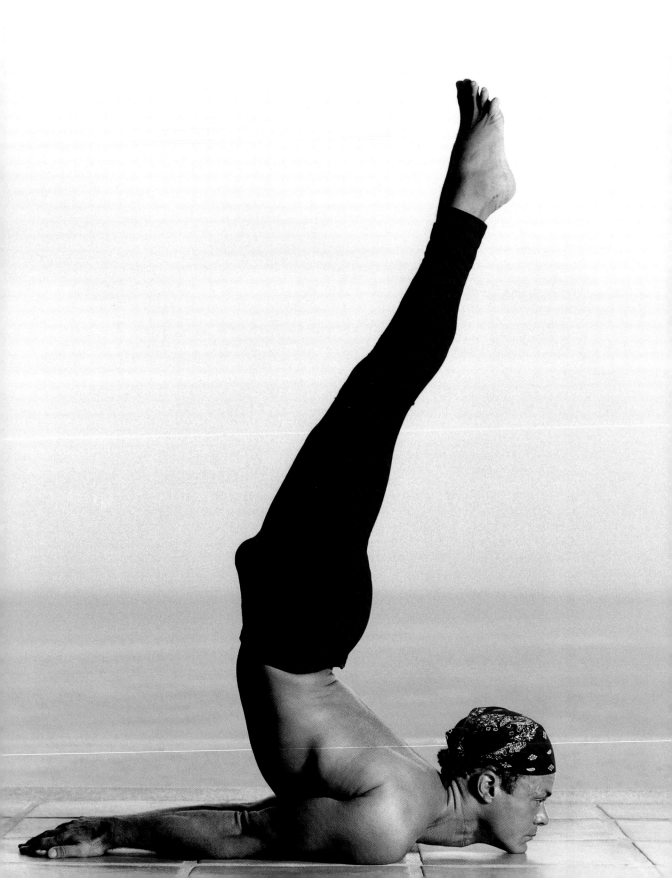

Tell me what you eat and I will tell you what
you are.

—Anthelme Brillat-Savarin

PART 3

The Cleansing

Diet

I FREQUENTLY GET ASKED, WHAT SHOULD I EAT? HOW MUCH SHOULD I EAT? WHAT IS THE "YOGIC" WAY TO EAT?

There are lots of "experts" who would be happy to answer this question, but I believe anyone can slap a universal diet on you and claim it will work absolutely. That's not what I'm here to do, and it certainly isn't what this program is about. We are each different, with unique tastes, digestive systems, metabolisms, and psychological and spiritual needs. Suggesting that everyone eat the same things or the same way is like saying we should all wear the same pants, even if they are too tight, too short, or are just completely not our style. Just like a yoga pose, no two authentic diets will ever look the same, nor should they. There are six billion people on this earth and each of us is unique.

Let me say this: You *don't* have to become a vegetarian to do yoga. You don't have to start drinking blue-green algae, or eating only raw foods, or fasting. These are all part of the dogma that surrounds a lot of yogic teachings, but from my perspective, it's more about personal truth than blindly following tradition. Gandhi was a vegetarian, but not arbitrarily; even he, for whom vegetarianism was a religious custom, experimented and researched other ways of eating until he chose from within his soul the way he should eat.

To me, it all comes down to eating consciously and cleanly. Eating clean isn't a requirement for having a yoga practice. But as you journey deeper into your power, you'll want to give up your negative eating habits.

When people commit themselves to living consciously and start to experience the positive, healthy changes in their bodies and their lives, they start to want to eat better, too. It just happens organically: Once you unveil your authentic mind, body, and spirit through rewiring your mind, practicing yoga, and meditating, growth becomes the main focus. You naturally want to awaken in all the areas of your life, and that includes what you eat. You start to want to show up on your mat and in your life cleaner and lighter. The energy of transformation spreads into every corner of your existence like healing sunshine. You start to look and feel better through the yoga practice, and suddenly the idea of greasy pizza and french fries is no longer appealing. You don't have to give up your cravings; they give you up instead. It sounds like magic, but it's true: I've seen it happen to countless people—myself included!

The problem is that there is so much conflicting advice about food out there that it's hard to know what to believe or even where to begin. You may have tried different diets and ended up abandoning them because they were too strict, too confusing, or just simply too alien. What went wrong was not understanding that these diets were only addressing a small fraction of your whole picture. The specifics of what you eat comprise the 20 percent technique I talked about earlier. You can try all the diets you want, but as I've said many times, the mechanics will always fail you without a shift in your underlying worldview. What really matters is changing the 80 percent psychology behind your relationship to food. And that key piece is the heart of my Cleansing Diet.

Your Relationship to Food

The power that food has over our minds is profound. In so many ways, Americans use food as a drug. In the best sense, our chemical and biological reactions to food fuel us and help our bodies function at peak performance. But so many Americans use this chemistry in the worst sense: as a drug to numb, comfort, distract, or take the edge off in moments of emotional distress.

So many of us fall prey to emotional reactiveness and then stuff ourselves compulsively. It is very common for people to eat when they become emotionally upset or nervous. When we get really stressed or frustrated, we hypnotically turn to food to alter our mood in that moment. Food can represent a way to fill the emptiness created by fear, anger, stress, sadness, or anxiety. We go unconscious to what and why we are overeating, and then wonder why we are a slave to our cravings. Food appears as a friend or solution in our moment of need, but many snacks later, it becomes apparent that the solution to the problem has become a problem in and of itself.

Years ago I had a student named Joe who was very overweight. Joe came to my studio in Philadelphia on the recommendation of his doctor, who himself was a student and suggested power yoga as a way for Joe to lose the weight that was endangering his health. For the first two months, Joe came pretty regularly, and I was surprised to note that his weight didn't appear to change at all. It is rare for people who carry extra weight not to lose it if they practice power yoga consistently.

After about three months, I started to notice a change in Joe. He looked like he had started to shed a few pounds, but more than that, he seemed different somehow— happier, a little lighter in energy. At the end of one class, Joe came over to me and offered me his thanks.

"You're very welcome," I said, assuming he was just thanking me for the class.

"No," Joe said. "I really want to thank you, not just for today. You said something a few weeks ago that made me think about the way I treat my body in a whole new way."

"What was that?" I asked.

"You said that to really heal, we need to be willing to feel. And I suddenly saw that all the diets I have tried are useless until I deal with the root of the problem—all the emotional stuff I've been cramming down."

Joe went on to tell me that he tried it my way just to see what would happen. The next time he had a bad day at work, instead of doing what he normally would, which was head to Mrs. Field's in the lobby of his office building and eat three chocolate chunk cookies and a large coffee with cream and extra sugar, he just stayed with the frustration. It wasn't easy, but he sat with it and didn't run from the pangs of anxiety in his chest. He suddenly realized that his bad days at work were really a result of being in the wrong place in his life. He was not living from his inner light. He wasn't being true to what was in his heart, and instead was dealing with his situation in a roundabout way. Joe saw how he had been cutting himself off from so many possibilities by always rushing to numb the discomfort. The shift of his intention to stay centered and allow his feelings to break through enabled Joe to see options where before he only ran for food. Within his pain was the message he needed in order to transform his life.

Healing comes in those moments when you look into your mind, observe your cravings, your excuses about eating in that moment, and are willing to let the real cause surface. You interrupt the negative pattern through being aware and start to create new wiring. Remember, there are two ways to heal any pain or anxiety: You can go the route of ego denial, indulging in food, drink, or cigarettes as a means of escape, which reduces you to a state of utter dependency. Or you can face the truth, admit your error, take your licks, feel, be sad, cry . . . let whatever is there come up and then let it go, which leads to genuine healing. The choice is always yours.

Just as when you hit your edge on the yoga mat, by not running away in the moment of anxiety or escaping into the arms of pseudo-comfort, you will probably feel old pains, anxieties, and guilt coming up to the surface to be resolved and released. These moments open a door in your mind to learning about yourself. Staying with the discomfort allows you to receive insights into how you have used food as a drug to soothe negative feelings. By feeling what is there in that moment, you heal not only your relationship to food, you also open the door to healing the underlying cause of the symptom.

The diet and guiding principles in this section will give you the tools to lose weight permanently, but ultimately, transformation in this area comes as a result of giving up the struggle, finding an inward surrender to the truth that will set your relationship to food free. Our relationship to food heals when we heal our emotional wounds, destructive lifestyle patterns, and our overreactions to everyday stress—all things that are illuminated as we commit to a truthful path.

Cleansing the Internal You

The cornerstone of the Cleansing Diet is the word *cleanse.* The entire Journey into Power life transformation program focuses on shedding the layers and blocks that hold you back, starting with those in the body. And if you're cleaning house in your body, doesn't it make sense to start with what you put into it? The Cleansing Diet is about transforming your relationship with food every day of your life.

Everything you eat is either fuel that sustains and energizes you, or a burden that clogs and drains you. The Cleansing Diet is about eating clean: taking into the body foods that nourish, replenish, and flush rather than pollute. It's really no more complicated than that. The simplicity of this process will make sense to you on a deep level, and your body will reward you in countless ways. From the moment you begin to "clean house" and rid yourself of even a small amount of toxins, waste matter, and metabolic debris stored in tissue and floating around in your bloodstream, you will begin to experience emotional and physical weight loss that creates a new vitality and clarity. Whatever it takes to restore your body to balance and bring it back to its ideal and authentic state, the Cleansing Diet will make it happen. Changes will happen quicker and easier than you think.

The Cleansing Diet is not a diet in terms of what we have come to think of as a "diet"; it's built on a foundation of universal and guiding principles that are timeless. By definition, universal means that they apply to any situation in relation to food. There are no recipes, no straitjacket regimens, no portion restrictions, no strict menus to follow. There are no absolute dos and don'ts. The Cleansing Diet isn't about what you eat at every meal, or how much, or when. It doesn't focus on restricting calories, fat, or carbohydrates. There is no color-coding, no pills, shakes, or potions. In fact, calling the Cleansing Diet a "diet" as we have come to use the word is somewhat misleading, because it is so much more than that: It's a principled, centered way of life. In fact, the word *diet* comes from the root *diaita,* which means "a manner of living." The Cleansing Diet is not an isolated element but rather an integral part of your whole Journey into Power.

There are two parts to the Cleansing Diet: the Guiding Principles and the Detoxifying Cleanse. The Guiding Principles are like true north on a compass— they always point you in the right direction so you'll intuitively know what is good for you and what is not. They bring you into alignment with nature's laws. They are based on psychological principles and physiological truths that guide you to your innate sense of how to fuel your body. These principles are so natural and potent that incorporating them into your system—and your life—will change your entire relationship to food and eating every waking moment of your life.

A powerful element of this program is to engage in the Detoxifying Cleanse, which is the seven-day detox we do at my Bootcamps. It is based on the idea that natural, spontaneous healing and purification can happen when you put your usual habits on hold while consciously focusing on eating for intensive cleansing. It gives you the chance to halt the cycle of negative eating habits and return your body to its normal state of balance and energy. In essence, it wipes the slate clean.

The reason the Guiding Principles come first is so you may understand the 80 percent psychology of this process. The Detoxifying Cleanse will boost your overall process, but the Guiding Principles are ultimately more important, because they are the philosophies and practices that will light your path, empower you, and allow you to establish the everyday eating rhythms that are natural and authentic to you.

I've seen the Cleansing Diet Principles radically affect thousands of my students. The ones who come to Bootcamps arrive tired, heavy in spirit, and sluggish, weighed down by stress and extra pounds. But seven days of potent and powerful yoga practice and eating clean gives their overtaxed, overstuffed digestive systems a rest, and as a result, they leave lighter, cleaner, and clearer. They have far more energy and a whole new perspective on food and eating. Many are so blown away by the effects of the Cleansing Diet Principles that they never go back to the unhealthy eating habits they brought with them the first night they arrived. They don't have to will themselves not to want sugar; their bodies automatically crave more healthful alternatives. Many are no longer ruled by the caffeine habit or the nicotine dragon, and are thus free from years of headaches, digestive problems, or long-term health dangers. Their desire for fresh, life-giving fruits and vegetables is sharpened, and their cravings for red meat and heavy dairy products fall away effortlessly. They naturally choose to adopt the principles of the Cleansing Diet into their lives once they experience what this level of detoxing does for them.

Not long ago, on one of those first evenings of a Bootcamp, I ran into a student on the beach path. There was something about him that was familiar, but I couldn't place his face. He clearly knew me and greeted me warmly. The guy laughed and said, "You don't recognize me, do you?"

"I'm sorry," I said. "You look familiar, but . . ."

"That's okay," he said with a grin. "That's actually a good thing. The last time you saw me was here, four months ago, at your last Bootcamp. I've lost thirty pounds since then."

With that information, I did recognize him and could hardly believe the transformation. When I saw him last he was bloated and overweight, with an unhealthy pallor. Now here he was, slim and fit and practically glowing—and it was only the first day of this Bootcamp! He told me that he had stuck with the daily power yoga, meditation, and the Cleansing Diet since returning home to Arizona, and the weight had just slipped away as though it never belonged there in the first place. I remem-

bered that he had told us at the previous Bootcamp that he had developed some terrible habits (having pizza and beer several times a week, eating frozen dinners and packaged snack foods, smoking) over the past year due to stress; it was great to see a freedom and lightness to him that had not been present before.

Certainly the outward results of eating cleaner are terrific, but they aren't the only reward. The transformation goes much deeper, and that's why the results are lasting. The Principles of the Cleansing Diet focus on *letting go* of the luggage of life: cleansing you from the inside out, beginning at the cellular level and then raising the altitude of your emotional and spiritual attitudes. You won't just feel better; you'll *be* better.

Here are only a few of the results you can expect from the Cleansing Diet:

The toxic debris that blocks your natural flow of energy will dissolve.

You'll shed unwanted fat, cellulite, weight, and inches if that's what needs to happen.

You'll put on healthy weight if that's what you need.

Your body will return to its authentic stature.

Your skin will radiate.

Stomachaches and intestinal problems disappear.

Your breath will be clean and sweet.

Problems like body odor, constipation, and general fatigue disappear.

You will have renewed energy and vitality.

Your emotions and moods will stabilize.

You will no longer have the midafternoon crash, when you look to a cup of coffee or sugary snack as a pick-me-up.
You will feel psychologically empowered, because you will have gained control over your eating habits.

Why not give these powerful and proven Cleansing Diet Principles a chance in your life? What do you have to lose besides excess fat, negative eating habits, and poor health? Whether you are looking to lose weight, gain weight, or achieve glowing health, you owe it to yourself to learn to eat consciously. As I always say, if not now, when?

The Cleansing Diet Guiding Principles

There are many natural laws of food and eating, but what I have done here is to boil them down to the most essential ones. You've probably had years of confusing diet advice thrown at you, and that's not what we're after here. We're looking to keep it simple, to pare it down to the basics and learn how to eat according to the natural wisdom already encoded within us.

You don't need to immediately incorporate all of these laws at once. Take your time with them. Experiment, hold them in your mind and incorporate them into your daily life in ways that work for you. As you peel away more and more of your layers, these laws will open the door to freedom from the negative eating habits that enslave

you. You will ultimately be empowered because you free yourself from feelings of guilt, shame, or remorse when it comes to your body and how you treat it. You will create a relationship to food, eating, and your body that fuels your highest potential.

If you apply the principles on a regular basis, the excess weight and baggage will vanish. Once you absorb this information, you will have at your fingertips unique tools to use whenever you feel unwanted symptoms sneaking back in.

Guiding Principle 1: Bring Mindfulness to Your Eating Habits

So many of us are in a food fog. We zone out when it comes to eating, robotically shoveling food into our mouths, often just because it's there. How many times have you automatically polished off a huge bag of buttered popcorn in the movie theater, simply because it's there in your lap? Have you ever stuffed yourself to capacity at a buffet, wondering afterward (as you clutch your aching gut) why you did that? Or found yourself standing in front of an open refrigerator door, vaguely searching for something to satisfy an even vaguer hunger? We go on autopilot, completely numb to what we are doing to ourselves.

The tragic truth is that most people treat their automobiles better than their own bodies. If it were proven that smoking cigarettes in a car would instantly corrode the engine, most every smoker would quit lighting up in his or her car. No automobile owner would pour a Coke into the gas tank, or stuff a fatty steak into the carburetor, or dump a banana split into the radiator. They would never damage their precious machines that way. They will put only the highest-quality fuel in their cars, routinely change the oil, and take their car in for tune-ups, like clockwork. Yet these same owners drive their precious cars up to the drive-in window of fast-food restaurants and wreak havoc on their physical machine!

Eating is an act of communion with the living forces of nature; it's where we take the power of Mother Nature into our bodies and spirits for nourishment. Sadly, because of the attitudes and habits most of us have learned about food, we often take it for granted. We forget that food is a precious gift. I have learned that when we forget food is a gift, it becomes a tyrant and betrayer. We go unconscious to it, ceasing to pay attention to the powerful effect it has on us. Depending upon our attitudes and awareness toward it, food is either a friend who supports us at every level or a fiend who can wreck havoc on our bodies and our lives.

I know firsthand how easy it is to be unconscious about what we eat. I have lived the Cleansing Diet Principles, which for me was just part of my upbringing, my entire life. Growing up in California in the sixties and seventies, I was greatly influenced by my surroundings: my parents' bustling yoga studio, health food restaurant, and traveling health and meditation

retreats. It was all I knew, and it was second nature to me, so it was easy to continue to respect these principles as an adult.

But in 1995 I threw myself into completely different surroundings. I moved from "organic" Los Angeles to "Cheese Steak Capital of the World" Philadelphia. I became the peak-performance specialist for the NFL's Philadelphia Eagles and started eating their traditional diet—full of fats, meats, dairy, chemically enhanced seasonings, soda, sports drinks, and so on. As you can imagine, between the food and the hectic schedule of professional sports, I quickly put on twenty pounds!

Because my job with the Eagles was to create peak performance, one of my first tasks upon joining the team (after realizing what their food was doing to them and to me!) was to change their diet. For the first time, the Eagles were cutting out fried foods, replacing fatty meats with lean proteins, skipping refined sugars and sweets. I witnessed it three meals a day when we would sit down and eat together. This was the year they made it to the playoffs ('95–'96).

Who can say how much the cleaner diet had to do with their performance? I don't presume to take credit for their success, but I did see the magic in the lives and bodies of these elite athletes. Many lost extra fat, replacing it with metabolically active bulk muscle. Most testified to the increase in energy and vitality they felt and the decrease in aches, pains, and tightness in their joints. If nothing else, my years of experience in the world of professional sports was one more testimony to and confirmation of the power of these yogic principles when authentically applied.

There is only one way out of the food fog, and that is to become aware and remain mindful of your relationship to food. It takes some practice to link your brain to what you eat, but here is where the mindfulness you learn on the mat can help you. Think back to what yoga is: the science of maximizing, refining, and improving your relationship to everything that is relevant to being alive and attaining your highest potential and purpose. When you consider that food is one of the most basic elements to life, you can see how vital it is that you pay attention to your relationship to it. It can either ruin or refine your existence here on earth. Food is *that powerful!*

Two of the most fundamental truths of yoga are mindfulness and intention. Both are hardly ever as important as when you are eating. Would you shovel in unhealthy food or monstrous portions if you were truly conscious of what you were doing? There are many ways to establish more awareness at every meal or snack. The following is a list of tools and awareness questions to bring more mindfulness to every bite you take. If you are ever truly going to find peace in your relationship to eating and food, mindfulness is a must!

1. Before you eat anything, always ask: Am I eating to escape, or to excel? Am I feeding my ego (to deny feelings and numb out), or am I nurturing my body? Is my eating a result of hunger, or to mask a deeper emptiness?

2. Observe a few moments of silence and give thanks for your food. Thankfulness is a profoundly spiritual act that will change your relationship to food significantly. Realize that food has the power to nourish your spirit as well as your body, and call forth gratitude for that gift. It is impossible to experience gratitude and be unconscious at the same time.

3. Listen to your body's signals. Can you detect when your body says, "enough"? Discovering and following your body's cues is the master key toward learning to eat mindfully.

4. Become aware of unhealthy cravings. Make a commitment to pausing between having a craving and automatically indulging it. Ask yourself, Where is this coming from? What do I really need? Often, if you interrupt the pattern with some movement, meditation, yoga, and/or a walk, you can redirect your focus and shift out of the craving or need.

5. Try preparing food consciously. Can you be totally present and mindful while peeling, chopping, mixing, and cooking? Can you really notice the colors, textures, and tastes? Being conscious around food, even the preparation of it, is a powerful force in transforming your attitude to it.

6. Become aware of the atmosphere in which you eat. Do you eat on the run, while working or watching television? Or do you

take the time to sit down and relax while you are eating? What effect do both scenarios have on your digestion? Eating while you are tense, upset, or agitated tends to trigger negative symptoms in your digestive tract. Eating in a calm, quiet atmosphere, however, sets a relaxed tone for healthy digestion.

7. Bring awareness to what you add to your food (dressing on your salad, sugar in your coffee, butter on your bread). These elements often go unnoticed, but they add up. A student named Elena once told me that when she was younger she noticed that her father added huge spoonfuls of white sugar to his tea every day. So she challenged him to put a spoonful of sugar into an empty soup bowl each time he put a spoonful in his tea. At the end of the week, he was shocked to see that it was almost overflowing! Try Elena's method and see how much sugar and fat you add to your diet without even noticing.

8. Do you have indigestion, gas, and gastrointestinal strain after you eat? Can you relate these symptoms to the foods you are eating or the combinations in which you are eating them? Attributing stomach problems to what, when, and how much you eat enables you to start regulating more consciously.

9. Pay attention to how your body feels in the minutes and hours after you eat. Are there foods that make you feel tired? Foods that make you feel light? Start relating your bodily sensations to what you've eaten to establish the cause-and-effect links

in your mind. Again, listen for internal cues.

Bringing consciousness to what and how you eat is the magical solution to changing your eating habits. Every bite you take with mindful awareness sets off another spark that lights the way out of the food fog.

Guiding Principle 2: Eat Intuitively

Have you ever tried a fad diet? Be honest. Have you ever sworn off all carbs including bananas and carrots but gobbled bacon and eggs, drank chalky pseudochocolate shakes, replaced lunch with a "dietetic" snack bar, or believed a television commercial that promised eating a sandwich every day from a fast-food sub shop could lead to miraculous weight loss? If you have, you're certainly not alone. Americans spend billions of dollars a year on weight-loss schemes, but the sad truth is that none of them ever work. That's why there is a new one every year! Even if you do manage to take weight off, you most likely gain it right back as soon as you stop following the program.

The reason none of these programs works is simple: They aren't real. Diets are a huge hoax! They aren't based on feeding our authentic bodies the way nature intended. They're based on techniques that defy the instinctive, healthy way our bodies need and process food.

We have been listening to the din of so many "expert opinions" that our own inner voice of wisdom has been drowned out. If you look to outside sources for what and how to eat, you'll just be eating according to someone else's idea of what is good for you. Of course, there are sensible basics of human nutrition that many experts speak about, but if you tune in, you'll find that you already know what you should and should not put into your body. On some deep level (perhaps so deep that it is still hidden to your conscious mind), you know what your body needs in order to function at its peak-performance level. We're genetically encoded with that wisdom. It's not that you need someone else to tell you; it's that you need to tune in and train yourself to hear the voice of your own intuition. There's a big difference between honestly educating yourself about food and listening to what experts have to say and blindly accepting everything you learn without questioning whether it makes sense to you.

The key to tuning in to your eating intuition is to *eat from cause*. What does it mean to "eat from cause"? It means that before you put anything into your body, you stop and ask yourself a simple question: What will this food *cause* in me? Will it produce guilt, regret, bloating, stomach discomfort, fat? Or will it produce sustenance, energy, and overall good feelings about your power of choice? Will it deplete you or invigorate you? Will it create temporary satisfaction (good taste) but long-term remorse?

By pausing to ask this key question, you put space between the stimulus and response, which in turn allows you to make more conscious choices. You don't zoom directly from craving to indulgence; you experience the craving, pause to ask, What will this food *cause* in me?, then *choose* whether to indulge based on the answer. That's the first step in learning to eat consciously, from intuition. As time goes by, it becomes automatic, and you no longer have to feel trapped by your cravings because you're now flowing from an unconscious competence.

To intuit *what* to eat, you need to first key in to the foods that create pain in you—indigestion, fat, guilt, nausea, sluggishness—and the foods that create authentic pleasure—energy, lightness, and feeling cared for in a healthy way. From there, you find the flow by creating balance between the two. If you overindulge in foods that cause pain, counterbalance by sticking with pleasure foods for a few days. Conversely, if you have eaten cleanly for a good stretch of time, you can indulge a bit.

This balance is important for two reasons: first, for psychological purposes, so you don't feel as if you're in a straitjacket, and second, because your body instinctively protects itself by storing fat, in case of deprivation (harkening back to cavemen days). If you constantly rein it in too tightly, it receives the signal "Uh-oh, no more food . . . better store up!" If your body receives a signal of sufficiency, however, it won't store up fat. None of this is about never eating the foods you love. If you love sweets, you can work them in in a balanced way. It's not what you eat at every moment that necessarily matters. The key question is, really, What is dominating?

As your intuition about food and the effect it has on you matures, you'll eventually find the balance that is right for you. What works for me is to eat cleanly five days a week, then allow myself to relax and indulge a bit if I feel like it on the other two. Because my system is pretty clean overall, it can handle these two days. I don't go overboard, because after so many years of eating intuitively, I've stopped craving the really toxic stuff, but it's not a big deal if I do indulge once in a while. My boys love ice cream, and some of the happiest moments of my life have been just sitting around with them wearing ice cream on their faces and laughing and talking. Food can be one of the greatest connectors between people, and remembering to enjoy yourself around it is so essential to our mental well-being.

As for tuning in to *when* or *how much* your body needs to eat, Mother Nature provided us with a foolproof way of knowing the answer: hunger! Deciding if you're hungry is like deciding if you're in love. If you're not sure—you're probably not.

Pay attention. Are you hungry in the morning? Do your days run better if you eat fruit before noon? Do dairy products puff you up? Are you better off eating frequent small meals throughout the day

rather than three large ones? Throw out the rules that don't work for you and key in to what does. Remember, it's a process of refinement, and your intuition is always right. It's never ever wrong.

The catch, though, is not to fool yourself into thinking that something you want to be true really is true. In other words, if your ego is telling you that your life really does run better if you have a big hunk of chocolate cake for breakfast, you *should* question it. The key to knowing if it is your intuition or your ego talking is that when your intuition speaks, you feel at peace with your choice. If it's your ego talking, chances are you'll feel defensive, as if you need to somehow justify your choice. If you feel defensive about a food choice, question which part of you is really making that choice. When the choice is right, you will clearly be at peace.

Guiding Principle 3:
Discover Water-Rich Foods and
Learn Why Your Body Needs Them

Water is nature's cleanser. Drinking pure water is great, and you should drink plenty of it, but what I'm talking about here is the water content of your food. Water alone doesn't nourish the body or undo the effects of a gooey and gluey diet. The goal here is to maximize our energy, flush the gastrointestinal tract so that things keep moving, and help keep us as clean on the inside as possible.

A water-rich diet is easier on your digestive system, as water-based foods require much less energy to digest than those based on fat. Digestion is a huge energy drain on the body, and when your body does not need to keep those digestive fires roaring in overdrive, you experience an immediate lift in energy. Anyone who has ever skied a whole day knows this to be true. The first half of the day you feel pretty good, and if dressed properly you can stay relatively warm. Then you go have lunch, which in ski culture is usually a big heaping bowl of chili con carne or cream-based chowder, and when you go back out on the slopes, everything is just a little bit harder. You even feel colder, because your body is using all its energy to digest the heavy food, leaving little left over for warmth or athletic agility.

So the question is: What are high-water-content foods? Fresh fruits and vegetables and their *freshly squeezed* juices contain the most water and carry with them the most valuable nutrients for our systems.

The water found in fresh fruits and vegetables has a special quality. Unlike plain drinking water, the water from living foods contains enzymes and nutrients that are all transported into the intestinal environment where they are absorbed and used by the body. The two-part benefit here is that nutrient-rich waters are maximizing the vitality of the cellular environment to flush residue or metabolic leftovers and at the same time replenishing and enriching each cell.

Of all foods, fruit is the closest to nature: It is mostly water and takes the least amount of energy to digest. Eating fruit alone allows the body to cleanse. Once a month, I take a day of rest and just eat fruit all day long. I started doing this over twenty years ago and I believe it has greatly contributed to my health, energy, and vitality. When I lead Bootcamps and put everyone on three days of fruit only, the levels of energy and youthfulness go through the roof!

One student, Carmen, was pretty alarmed by the idea of the three-day fruit fast. She was worried that she would be hungry, that she would feel deprived and weak without protein. But she made it through, and on the last evening, when everyone was sharing their experiences, she stood up and showed us that her jeans were a few inches too loose on her.

"I could barely button these pants at the beginning of the week!" she said. "You all know how freaked out I was at first that I was only going to eat fruit for three days, but I can't believe how powerful I feel. It's amazing. All I could think about on the first day were cheeseburgers, but now I don't even want one if it means I'll be able to feel like this!"

What Carmen discovered was the same thing you will experience if you consciously replace heavy, carb-loaded, fatty foods in your diet with those that are water-rich: boundless energy, fewer unhealthy cravings, and an overall elevation of vitality. You don't need to do a total fruit fast to feel these results; even the slightest shift toward water-rich foods will make a difference.

If you'd like to ease into the benefits of fruit cleansing, try eating fresh fruit by itself in the morning. You will find it to be a solvent that acts as an internal flush. It also starts up your metabolic fires without clogging up your system. Remember, each night is a rest for your digestive tract. So you want to break your fast (break-fast) with foods that will begin your day in the cleanest way possible. Start weaning yourself from eggs, starches, processed cereals, bacon, sugary muffins, and other stuff with which you load your body at the beginning of your day, and I guarantee you will feel renewed energy and vitality.

From today forward, commit yourself to replacing the foods that create lethargy, fatigue, and sluggishness with those that nourish, cleanse, and remove the waste that blocks your energy. Before you put anything into your mouth, ask yourself: Will this food leave me feeling lighter or heavier? Will it cleanse me or clog me?

Guiding Principle 4:
Learn Why Trying to Fool Mother Nature Makes You a Fatter Fool

The most basic of all principles is simply getting back to nature and her life-giving foods. Today the health-conscious, fat-phobic people of this country are spending millions of dollars on diet foods that are highly processed, refined, preserved, and altered. America seems to be on a big low- to nonfat diet craze and yet she is fatter and more diseased than ever! Why? Because the nonfat foods we choose are artificially nonfat; they are basically fake foods. They are made of chemicals and additives—substances that poison your body and that your body cannot use or assimilate properly. Our bodies weren't created to metabolize artificial food. Eating fats that have been hydrogenated or chemically altered in a hundred other ways takes nature out of the equation and actually puts a huge strain on your body's metabolism and digestion. Eating artificially means eating sludge. Eating sludge drains energy, so you're less likely to move, digest, and eliminate. Not moving and not breathing makes you toxic, unhappy, fat, and depressed.

I remember when I was living in Los Angeles seeing people walk around with gigantic cups or cones of nonfat frozen yogurt. Most of these people were overweight and had bought into the scheme that just because something says it is nonfat means that it is good for you, or that you can eat as much as you want without having to worry about negative effects. It's exactly the opposite! People eat entire boxes of low-fat cookies—empty carbohydrates that turn to fat in your system, thinking they are doing their bodies a favor, when really all they are doing is loading their system with more artificial, health-robbing, fat-building waste.

Foods that are newly nonfat (meaning that something has been extracted from the food, thus changing the makeup of the food from what nature had intended) are as far from whole foods as you can get. Eating dead, processed, additive- and preservative-filled food means you are choosing to live in a lifeless, processed, added-to, and preserved body! Sounds like a processed corpse, doesn't it? Wouldn't it make more sense to eat living, whole, nutrient-rich foods instead?

Why do we presume that we can make foods better than the way they came from the earth? Mother Nature knew what she was doing when she created our original forms of sustenance. To eat organic, whole food, as close to the way it came from the earth as possible, means to keep yourself aligned with the power and force of nature. Living food is everything a creature needs. What do you think would happen if you fed a diet of cooked and candied straw to a horse, or eucalyptus strudel to a koala bear?

Make eliminating fake foods and chemicals from your diet your new life focus and you will feel the difference immediately. Your natural state of health is just that: natural. Eliminate preservatives, additives, artificial food colorings, and dyes. This includes MSG, extra sugars, corn syrups, artificial sweeteners, nitrates/nitrites, olestra or other fake fats, imitation flavorings, and so on. By taking these fake substances out of your diet, you will lose inches, lethargy, and prevent or reverse disease. You will add years to your life and life to your years.

Here are some ideas for how you can move yourself toward clean foods while easing yourself away from pollutants:

- Buy food brands that are chemical-free (remember, chemicals in your food become chemicals in your body). Your local health food store is the best place to find tasty, chemical-free alternatives.
- Eat food with the fewest ingredients possible. *Read labels!*
- Give up what I call "white death": white flour and white sugar. Choose instead whole grains and food sweetened with natural sweeteners.
- Use fresh and natural dressings, condiments, and seasonings (such as garlic, basil, onions, oregano, cumin, cinnamon, all-natural ketchup and mustard, etc.).
- Go for food in its natural state. This means avoiding boxed, canned, or pre-prepared foods.

Simply put, move yourself toward making better, cleaner, more natural food choices. Decide what is the right way for you as an individual to do this. For instance, you may never want to give up butter or other dairy products. But at least start to buy it in its organic form. My son and I love sausage, so I've opted to buy free-range, organic turkey sausages rather than the nitrate/nitrite-filled pork varieties. My eldest son loves pizza, but he's a vegetarian who doesn't eat cheese. So he either peels it off at birthday parties or we order pizza with sauce and toppings only. I think for any "tradition" to last and become part of us, we need to be free to choose how and what works for us.

Before you put anything in your mouth, ask yourself, How close to the earth is this food that I am about to eat? Is it whole or processed, real or fake?

Guiding Principle 5: Learn How to Live to One Hundred by Eating Less

Andrea was seriously into weight-lifting before she came to a Bootcamp. Everything she had read detailed that high-protein diets were the way to build muscle mass, so she was eating lots of protein at every meal. She would begin her day with an eight-egg-white omelet and continue eating five large meals throughout the day, convinced she needed the extra food to sustain her energy. When she heard she was going to do a weeklong Detoxifying Cleanse, she was skeptical but willing to try it.

Here is how Andrea described the experience:

"Day one of the Bootcamp, I was sure I was going to starve to death! I piled two, three plates high with the salads and fruits. People looked at me strangely, but I really believed that I needed to overeat in order to sustain my energy for all the yoga. As the week went on, the healthy and clean food filled me, and I began to see that I didn't need to eat so much. By the time the three-day fruit fast began (in the middle of the week), I was already eating about half

as much as I was on day one. The detox process was amazing to me—almost indescribable. I started to actually be able to taste how good the simple foods were. It was so clean and delicious, and I started to really understand that I only needed to eat small amounts to get full and to have tons of energy. Bootcamp changed my eating habits—and my life—forever!"

We are a culture of overeaters, trained by admonishments like "Don't let that go to waste" and "Clean your plate." We're not stuffing our faces because we're afraid there won't be any food tomorrow. We're stuffing our faces either because that is what we were taught to believe we must do or, in the case of emotional eating, to numb out.

Experts in cardiovascular disease estimate that at least one fourth of all heart disease problems can be attributed to overeating, which forces the heart and lungs to work harder than is healthy and become old before their time. Scientists who have studied the lifestyle of centurions attribute their long life to sparse eating habits. "Undereating" is something almost all of them have in common. Since they do not overtax their bodies and digestive systems, they just last longer. As Ben Franklin said hundreds of years ago, "To lengthen thy life, lessen thy meals."

If you like to eat a lot, eat less at each meal and you'll end up eating more in the long run. How? Because you'll live longer if you eat less, and the longer you live, the more food you'll get to eat. A healthy eighty-year-old man certainly gets to eat a whole lot more than a man who dies at sixty from a heart condition brought on by obesity!

Eat less than you think you need to and, like Andrea, you'll be amazed at how much you were cramming into your body that you didn't need. Identify your true feelings of hunger and pay attention to when you reach the point of nonhunger (rather than feeling full). This doesn't mean skipping meals. It means eating smaller meals. Small meals throughout the day are like kindling—they keep the digestive fires burning. Large meals are like big heavy logs that consume the whole flame and reduce it to smoldering smoke.

I eat five to six small meals throughout the day, at least one or two of which I make in the blender. Fruit and protein powder shakes (I like whey protein) are a great source of energy without being a burden on the digestive system. You'll have to experiment on your own to see how often and how much you need to eat.

By eating less, I don't necessarily mean fasting. Some people are proponents of fasts, and if you are drawn to that, by all means research ways to do it healthfully and try it. But I believe if you live your life clean, you don't necessarily need to. I used to fast every Monday when I was younger, but it's not something I do anymore. Fasting can make your nervous system feel ungrounded and a little raw. I was younger then, with fewer responsibilities, and I think the more pressures you have in your life and the more urban environments you travel in, the more your nervous system needs to be grounded.

By eating less and eating clean, your yoga practice will soar, because you'll have better elimination, less weight, and more energy in general, rather than wasting your inner force on the digestion of excess food. Your life both on and off the mat will take on a whole new energy.

The Detoxifying Cleanse

Why detox?

Body toxicity is the root cause of many ailments we humans suffer. No matter how healthy you profess to be, no matter what measures you take to remain healthy, an ever-increasing level of toxicity will in time take its toll. Symptoms will accumulate and years of poor eating and other bad habits will gradually chip away at your immunity, vitality, and energy.

There is an experiment that shows that if you drop a frog into a pot of boiling water, he will jump right out and save himself. But if you put a frog into a pot of cool water and gradually heat it up to boiling, the frog won't notice and will boil to death. It's morbid but true. We're like those frogs, gradually turning up the heat on ourselves but never noticing because we have grown accustomed to the temperature. We're so used to how we feel, even when depressed, that we don't remember that vitality is an option.

Your body is always in a state of change, like a river. You can never step in the exact same river twice, because the currents are always moving and the water that was there just moments ago is already downstream. The location and name of the river may be the same, but the reality of it has changed. Your body is an active field of energy—each day it is being reconstructed, renewed, and replaced by new cells. It may look the same, but it is in a constant state of change. Detoxifying is a way to immediately direct that process of change toward a brighter destiny.

The mechanics of this are pretty simple. Once you get the junk out of your system, you stop craving it. You see and feel the results immediately and experience a lightness like never before. You've jammed a stick into the unconscious cycle of craving/indulging and enabled your system to begin dictating what your body really needs and wants instead of what your ego has fooled you into believing you want. I'm not promising that once you detox your system you'll never crave chocolate—or threatening that you can never have it again. This isn't about deprivation; it's about finding balance. (But I would be surprised if you found that your old cravings have the same appeal.) You'll be more attuned to your needs and be able to start eating from choice rather than feeling helpless to fight off your cravings.

Making the shift from unconscious to conscious eating is a significant transition, so you will probably experience some physical reactions along the way. If you are used to eating big, heavy meals, you may feel a little lightheaded at first as your body's energy is released from the burden of overtaxing digestion. If you are accustomed to the superficial energy from white sugar and caffeine, you will realize how tired you really are, and see how much you need to take care of your body. You might experience bad breath, irritability, and so on as the toxicity passes through your system. All these symptoms are completely normal. If these or similar symptoms arise, *do not worry!* They are all signs that your body is detoxing. Simply increase your intake of water and water-rich foods. Like any other pains of purification, they pass in time—usually within a few hours or days.

It takes energy for your body to work in its intensive healing and cleansing mode (also known as a "healing crisis"), so you may feel tired for a few hours or even a couple of days. If that's the case, give yourself some extra rest. Know that this lethargy will soon be replaced with radiant energy!

I urge you to take the time beforehand to set yourself up right. You can maintain your regular life, but try not to schedule any major events that week and to spend as much time as possible resting, practicing yoga, and being in nature. Trying to do a detox in the midst of a hectic schedule is like trying to meditate on the median of an eight-lane highway. It's better to create the optimum conditions rather than stack the odds against yourself.

Isn't your health and longevity worth a seven-day time out? Wouldn't you give seven days to have more energy, shed symptoms, and walk more lightly through life?

Seven Days That Will Last a Lifetime

The following seven-day plan progresses gradually. It begins with two full days of a modified macrobiotic diet, then moves into three days of fruit only, then comes back to a more regular eating plan for the last two. Throughout, we eliminate caffeine, alcohol, refined sugar, dairy, and artificial foods altogether. There are no strict guidelines as to how much or when to eat; use what you have learned in the Guiding Principles to determine that for yourself.

Days One and Two:

Your diet for these two days should consist of organic fresh fruits and vegetables, whole grains, and tofu, chicken, or fish. Here is a breakdown of what we usually eat at Bootcamp, which you can modify to accommodate your tastes:

Upon Awakening: One large glass of hot purified water with one half of a fresh lemon squeezed into it. You may add honey to sweeten if you wish. This tonic helps flush waste matter from your digestive tract and keeps your breath sweet.

Breakfast: Fresh fruit and freshly squeezed fruit juice, organic yogurt (if you eat dairy), chopped almonds to sprinkle in the yogurt or over sliced fruit, and as much

herbal tea as you want. You can use a little organic honey for sweetener.

Lunch: One serving of protein (tofu, fish, or skinless chicken breast), steamed, poached, or baked with no oil, and one serving of a whole grain (like brown rice). I usually equate one serving to one fist-sized portion of food. You may also have as much fresh vegetables and salad as you would like. You can use vinegar and lemon with one teaspoon of olive oil for dressing and natural seasonings as you wish. Make lunch your largest meal. But remember, less is more.

Snack: Any form of fresh fruit or vegetable.

Dinner: One serving of protein as at lunch and one serving of a whole grain and one serving of a vegetable or a salad. We usually have something different at dinner than at lunch for variety. For dessert, you can either have fresh or baked fruit, or you can get creative and make naturally low-fat, whole-grain, dairy-free desserts that you can get from any good vegan cookbook.

Days Three, Four, and Five:

Here is when you enter your three-day fruit fast. It sounds hard, but after two days of already eating light, it won't be as difficult as you think. You can have as much fresh, whole fruit or freshly squeezed juice as you want. Be creative! Instead of just eating an apple, or a pear, take the time to prepare a beautiful fruit salad that combines several kinds of fruit. Here are a few creative suggestions the chefs at our Bootcamps have come up with to make fruit a little more interesting:

Mash up a few bananas and freeze to make banana "ice cream."
Bake apples, using honey or cinnamon for flavoring.
Poach pears and use a little honey or cider for sweetening if you wish.

Remember, avocados and tomatoes are fruits, so you can use them to make soups, salads, guacamole, and so on. You can add a little tomato salsa (as long as there are no onions in it, because onions are not a fruit) or apple cider vinegar for flavoring.

Days Six and Seven:

For the last two days of your cleanse, you will go back to what you ate on Days One, Two, and Three. However, it is very important that you remain conscious of what you are doing. Your system is cleaner and lighter than it was three days ago, so you will probably need less food than you think you do. Stay conscious and present to what your body needs, referring back to the Guiding Principles of eating intuitively and bringing mindfulness to your eating habits.

Also:

- Practice yoga daily to help the cleansing process along—do at least thirty minutes of vigorous postures.

- Sweat every day (sauna, hot bath, hot yoga practice, aerobic exercise).
- Sleep at least seven to nine hours each night—your body is going through an energetic process and needs to rejuvenate.
- Do not deprive yourself of a meal or snack if you are hungry. Eating is necessary, natural, and good for you. Your metabolism needs fuel. Don't eat if you aren't hungry, as this will defeat the purpose of becoming aware of your hunger patterns.
- Attempt to detox your mind and emotions. *Meditate!* Rest or fast from excess news, television, and anything else that is overstimulating. Especially make your mornings and evenings as quiet, relaxing, and calming as possible. This process is for you, so take it as a form of retreat.
- Absorb the Guiding Principles so you can start preparing yourself for when the seven days are over.
- Enjoy yourself daily—commit to doing at least one thing every day for the next seven days that will bring a smile to your face.

Ending the Seven-Day Detox

At the end of the seven days, *do not* break your detox fast foolishly. The minute they wake up on the eighth day some people rush right out to have something that has been off-limits. That is the *worst* thing you could do to your system. Your intestines can't take that kind of shock. Believe me, I speak from experience. Years ago I did a ten-day detox fast, and at the end of it I ate a huge bag of raw cashews. Not just a handful or two, more like a pound or something. Needless to say I ended up curled in the fetal position, clutching my stomach for three days. It took my system weeks to recover from that shock, and trust me, I never did anything like that again. Any fool can fast, but only a wise person knows how to break it responsibly.

Modify your way out of a detox fast slowly. Give your system a chance to get regulated. You moved out some metabolic toxins over the past seven days; don't throw away all that effort just to strain and overload your system all over again.

I recommend doing this seven-day Detoxifying Cleanse to jump-start and boost your everyday Cleansing Diet, and then again a few times throughout the year, whenever you feel you have gone off track or just need to do a little internal clearing.

As we clean our physical house and remove that which blocks the natural functions of the body, the body's own wisdom can do its magic. The body's ability to restore itself is profound. As we free up the energy flow, we come into a new state of aliveness. Giving our systems a rest and fueling them with power rather than poison allows the body to go to work to heal, balance, and enjoy peak performance, both on and off our mats every day of our lives.

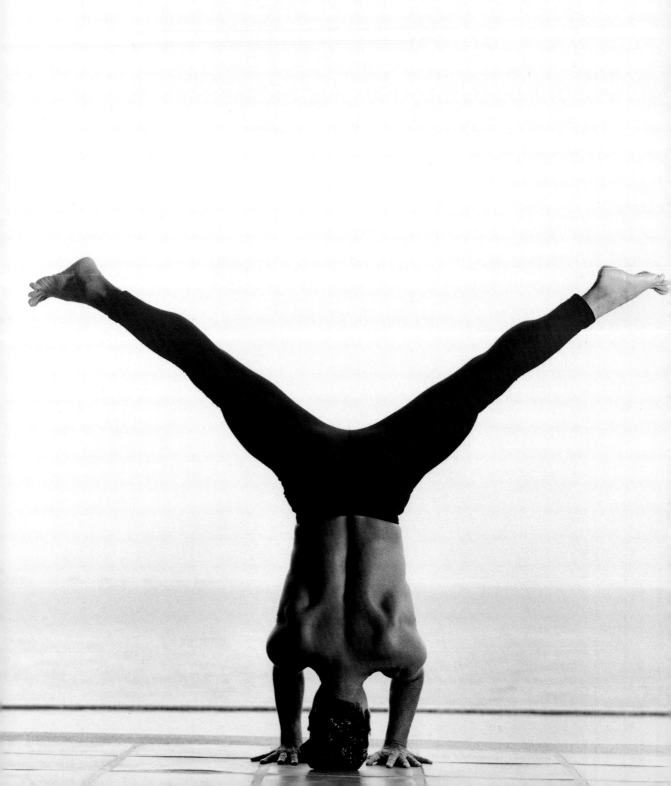

In order to be truthful you must embrace your total being.

—Rumi

PART 4

Meditation for
Truthful Living

WHAT DO YOU THINK OF WHEN YOU HEAR
THE WORD *MEDITATION?*

SWAMIS IN CAVES ON THE TOP OF A MOUNTAIN? PEOPLE SITTING IN

cross-legged positions for hours, chanting? Listening to a guided imagery tape telling you to envision yourself in some peaceful, exotic location?

For some people, this is meditating. But to me, meditating is not about how or where you sit or what you imagine. It is about anchoring your consciousness to the present moment, being fully awake in your body, aware of your thoughts, and surrendering to stillness. The purpose of meditation is simply to cultivate a quiet consciousness from which your emotions and intellect can flow.

We are always doing, doing, doing, and so it is a huge shift for us to suddenly do nothing. But if we successfully do nothing, something happens to us on a deeper and more profound level. We learn to be at ease in our own skin. We empty our emotional cups, clear the static from our mental attic, and open our minds and hearts so that we may see and live from our truth.

A lot of students tell me they can't meditate. Some say they've tried it and nothing happens. Others tell me they don't have the patience. Still others claim they don't have the time. But if you've started doing yoga, you've already begun the process of quieting your mind. Yoga and meditation go hand in hand—one practice enhances the other. You come into quietness through the practice of yoga, but you cultivate a connection to the guiding stillness within you through the practice of meditation.

I believe meditation can work for anyone if the intention is right. Certainly a beautiful, strong body and calm mind are wonderful things to cultivate, but if we seek these things by themselves, we are playing small. Playing at the highest levels involves having an honest, sincere intention to grow and a yearning to know the truths that can set us free. A pure intent awakens us to a new level of awareness that ultimately yields true and everlasting power.

Gaining a New Vantage Point

I'm not sure where I heard this, but there is a story about a man who bought a painting at a garage sale. It was a smallish canvas that was painted all gray. Everyone else thought it was ugly and bleak, but for some reason he was drawn to it. The frame was cracked, so he brought the painting in to a frame shop to get a new one. When the framer took the canvas out from the original frame, he discovered that it was folded over many times and was actually an enormous canvas. The gray spot was a cloud floating in a brilliant blue sky!

Meditation helps you cultivate what I like to call your "blue sky mind." It lets you take a step back from the center of your circumstances and gain a new vantage point. If you are lost in your head, you can

only see what is right in front of you. You are focusing only on the gray cloud. But when you take a step back, you can see the bigger picture. It can be a huge relief. It's very freeing to suddenly see that there's really lots of blue sky, and that all the junk going on in life is really just the clouds.

When we meditate, our brains emit different brain waves, creating new fields of consciousness and making space in our minds to receive new information and insights. Then when you go back to your everyday problems, you have uplifted your consciousness to a new place from which you'll have a clear perspective on how to let those problems fall away. You create some space—a little gap between stimulus and response. In that space, options arise. To the degree that you raise the altitude of attitude, the wider that gap becomes, and suddenly you are able to gain control over your circumstances instead of the other way around.

Do you know the peace and serenity you feel when you are on vacation? Three days on the beach, in the mountains, or on the road and suddenly your problems back home seem small and weightless. You can hardly remember why you were so stressed out. You swear you aren't going to get caught up in all the nonsense again, but within hours of arriving home the old dynamics surface and your temporary peace goes to pieces.

With meditation, though, the "vacation effect" can be long lasting, even permanent. In a way, every meditation is like a mini-vacation away from the conscious-ness in which you live. The calming effects are cumulative, and, over time, you live more consistently from the stillness of your soul.

When you meditate, the problems you brought with you are still there at the end of your practice—just like they are still there when you arrive home from vaca-tion. What has changed is your perspec-tive. You are given a new vantage point. Suddenly you can see solutions where be-fore you only saw problems, inspiration where before you could only perceive con-fusion.

On your yoga mat you begin to learn to halt the cycle of reactiveness, and a regular meditation practice deepens that aware-ness and takes it to the next level. When we overreact we lose our center of equilib-rium. But when difficulties and challenges arise, meditation teaches you to flow and function from a calm mind. While every-one else is in a panic, you stay centered and clear-headed. Meditation is the process of diminishing our reactions. It shows us that it is the way we respond emotionally to pressures that makes us either better or bitter. This remarkable process leads us back to our center of dignity and under-standing and gives us the ability to main-tain sanity and serenity no matter what is happening around or to us.

Russell, a student of mine, is the editor of a well-known monthly magazine. He and his staff thrived on pressure, and the week before every deadline would invari-ably be frenzied and stressful. There would be constant crises—articles not fin-ished, photos that still needed permissions, quotes that needed to be verified—and Russell usually spent one week out of every month living off Excedrin and Taga-met. Normally an even-tempered guy, he would get reactive and angry and would snap at his staff and his family until the magazine went to press.

At some point Russell started a regular meditation practice, and the very first month into his practice, he noticed that the week before deadline wasn't quite as bad as it usually was. At first he wasn't sure if it had anything to do with him; he thought maybe it was just an easier issue. But with each successive month, Russell would get calmer as the people around him got more panicked. He felt inspired rather than constricted and was able to find creative solutions where before everything seemed complicated and difficult to fix. It became clear that he had widened the gap in his normal stimulus/response cycle.

Russell no longer dreads the week be-fore deadline. He knows that he can now choose how he responds to circumstances that arise, and that whether his experience is a stressful or peaceful one is entirely within his power.

Control vs. Surrender

It seems that more and more people are looking to live from a simpler, truer, and more authentic place within themselves. So how do they accomplish this? By relinquishing control and learning to surrender.

The inner environment is not something we shape. It is something we must surrender to. The act of inner surrender is actually 180 degrees from the idea of self-mastery (or blindly following a teacher). It is a surrender to *your own intuition* and a willingness to act on that inner guidance as it comes to you.

One of the appeals that is often sold to us by many yoga and meditation teachers is that the practitioner can learn to master themselves or attain perfect self-control. This "spiritual" notion is actually ego-driven by its very nature; it teaches one to control and master his own fate, instead of being an open vessel to receive the guidance of the universe. This eventually inspires feelings of guilt and defectiveness in the person who doesn't quite hit the elusive mark of total self-mastery. For the perfectionist or Type A personality, this is like holding out the carrot at the end of a stick. It's a goal that you can never quite reach and that inevitably drives the groove of self-doubt even deeper.

Yoga and meditation for self-mastery says, "Don't come as you are, come as you are supposed to be." It's all about the goal of trying to become different or somehow better than you are. But I always tell my students, "Come to class as you are, not as you are supposed to be." Personally, I am opposed to the idea of self-mastery. For me it was a trap that took me many years to escape from. I still have some emotional

scars to remind myself of the hidden dangers of such a delusion.

About eighteen years ago I thought I had nearly mastered the kriya breathing technique of meditation, which is an intense form of psychic-mental concentration in which attention is shifted through various parts of the body. I remember one particular day of meditation at the ashram where I was living in Southern California. I had been practicing steadily for nearly nine hours and was so exhausted I could hardly continue breathing. A sense of utter failure suddenly overwhelmed me. After all my years of meditation training, I tasted a bitter defeat in the realization that I had still not "arrived."

In that moment of personal helplessness I was struck with the beautiful revelation that of myself I can do nothing, that all I really needed to do was stop trying so hard and surrender to a force within me that was greater than myself. I saw the fallacy of presuming that sheer strength of will and technique could catapult me beyond the confines of my own mind. Surprisingly, this breakthrough did not come through any superhuman effort or perfection of technique on my part, but rather as a result of my *abandoning* effort and technique. I got it firsthand that technique and willpower would always fail me and that it was an expansion and shift in my psychology that would ultimately set me free.

Seven years of full-time effort in meditation led to that moment in my life when I was finally forced to let go. I realized without a shadow of a doubt that a person cannot storm the gates of heaven through effort. In that moment of surrender I had become aware of an interior power—my intuition—that had been there all the time. Somehow and somewhere along my journey through life I had lost the connection I once had with this important part of myself. It was not until years later that I fully understood the dimension and significance of what had happened that day at the ashram, or that I would be fully able to process and interpret the depth of my experience.

After that revelation, meditation took on a whole new meaning for me. It became not about willpower or extreme effort but about surrender to the here and now by simply being awake, fully present in my body, and having the sincere intention for growth. Meditation became for me a practice of acceptance. Rather than using all my personal force to try to attain something I didn't have, the whole thrust shifted to simply accepting more deeply a power that I already had within me.

Some people call the experience I had enlightenment. The yoga community would call it cosmic consciousness, or samadhi. There are many labels for what happened, but I never felt the need to call it anything special. I didn't want to rob it of its simplicity and turn it into some ego-driven triumph. I didn't even feel the need to talk about it, because it felt so natural and fulfilling just to live the experience and its effects.

I have been surprised over the years to discover that this is not an uncommon happening. I have been contacted by many sincere people who have related their own experiences with meditation. Among them were a medical doctor, a Ph.D. student from Harvard, a full-time mother of four, prison inmates who have worked with my meditation CD, and literally hundreds of others who have told me about this new-found state of oneness within themselves. This story in particular stands out in my mind:

A woman named Emily who attended one of my teacher-training Bootcamps was going through a lot of marital difficulties. She and her husband of eight years had tried everything, including marriage counseling, but they were still stuck. So she had decided to get a divorce.

In the midst of this marital turmoil, Emily attended the Bootcamp and learned the meditation technique I will teach you here. Several months later she contacted me and said, "I continued to meditate as you taught us, and something just clicked inside me." She went on to say that she had canceled the divorce proceedings even though she was the one who had initiated them in the first place.

"Why?" I asked.

"Meditating just awakened all these amazing strengths and resources inside me," she explained. "I can now recognize my side of things. I see that the wisdom I need in our marriage will continue to come and guide me."

A couple of years later, Emily told me that she and her husband had resolved most of their major difficulties. She admitted that they still had their share of problems, but says she can now meet these challenges with greater clarity, calm, and inner strength.

I'm not promising that if you surrender to intuition you will automatically experience a great spiritual awakening. Perhaps you will, or perhaps you will receive other insights that will be personally profound. What I can promise you, though, is that pursuing self-mastery assures that you will never "arrive." In fact, there is no place at which to arrive, for you are there already. Your greatest power is not going to be here at any time in the future any more than it is already here right now. It's within you if you are just willing to relax, look inward, trust, and surrender.

Opening Your Heart to the Truth

Meditation is about lifestyle. It is a spiritual practice that leads you into the depths of your heart and soul so that you can live from within that zone in every moment. It is about mindfulness: being in the here and now, present to what is in front of you without trying to change it. It is an opening to what is true for and about you, having the courage to be honest and be who you are in every moment, to follow your heart, to listen to and act on the promptings of your own intuition. The more we listen to and trust what comes from

within, the stronger this relationship becomes. We start to know it as grace. Even a few minutes of meditation practice every day sets you on the road to truthful living. The technique I have practiced and taught for years is profoundly simple, and gradually becomes even simpler as you progress. Meditation gives you so little to do that your ego may find it difficult, even unacceptable. Its simplicity is unbearable to an ego that thrives on constant challenge and struggle! The results, on the other hand, are so profound that we tend to interrupt the process and spoil everything by trying to explain, label, or analyze it. The irony is that the less we do on the level of the ego, the more magic we will receive from this simple practice.

I'll go through the method a little later in this section, but suffice to say that it doesn't involve a whole lot more than just sitting quietly, being fully present, and observing your thoughts. By stepping outside your thoughts long enough to observe them, you begin to see that you are not your thoughts. This then helps you identify and strengthen the essential "you" within, the observer of the thoughts. It is very freeing to realize that your thoughts are separate from you, because as negative thoughts arise, you will be able to detach and release them as unwanted debris. Meditation hones your ability to dissolve festering thoughts and emotions one moment at a time.

What really matters, as always, is not so much the technique but the stuff that comes up around the practice and the willingness to deal with what is really in your heart. As you sit, the interior eyes of your mind turn 180 degrees, and suddenly you see things that you didn't even know were there: emotions, anxiety, resentments, trauma, beliefs, anger, grief . . . stuff that may be just beneath the surface and begging for release. Those truths may not always be pretty, but as it says in the Bible, "The truth shall make you free."

It can be painful to reveal the truth, so what do most of us do? As soon as we feel a little discomfort we try to get rid of it. We drink something, we eat something, we smoke something, we watch something, we have sex . . . anything to take away the pain of the moment. We are so busy looking for the way out of whatever ails us that we don't realize that the way out isn't an exit at all. The way out is reached by going in. Within us are the truths that can free us from the pain. They are locked within the chambers of our own hearts, yearning to come forth. And if you would just turn off the TV, put down the newspaper, unplug the phone, or close the refrigerator door, those truths could surface for release.

For me personally, meditation has a lot to do with slamming on the brakes of life and allowing myself to feel and see and be with what's there. That can be hard. I may not always like what I see or feel, but when I can look at something about myself I don't like without reacting to it, and accept it for what it is, that is the beginning of getting over it. I don't always practice this perfectly, but I try my best, and when I do, magic happens. My friend Jessie Peterson has taught meditation to some of the most prominent people in the world. One of the many things he teaches that I love is the idea that meditation introduces the "real you" to the "not you," so you can begin to distinguish one from the other. We are in many ways living in a state of hypnosis. We buy into the illusion that what we do and have is "us." Meditation helps us wake up to the reality of who we are without the doing and having. You dispel the illusion of who you thought you were by coming face-to-face with your authentic self.

I believe there is a ring of fire that we all must pass through as we exit the ego realm and come into the realm of the spirit. That is the collective pain and fear that has been a result of your history, your autobiography, and your unconscious patterns. Up to a certain point in our lives we live out our unconscious programming, and then we eventually come to realize that that programming isn't helping us reach our highest potential. The ring of fire is what separates the "real you" from the "not you," and meditation is the bridge across.

Emptying Your Daily Cup

Do you shower every morning?

My guess would be that you probably wake up and wash off the soot and grime of the previous day so you can start the new day clean and refreshed. It's second nature to most of us. We don't even think about whether or not we are going to wash the outside of our bodies; we do it automatically.

But how many of us cleanse our minds every morning? How many of us wake up each day and truly honor the needs of our spirits? How many of us crash into our day to the sound of a blaring alarm clock, or a rushed morning routine, or the violence and depressing news reported in the morning paper? What do *you* feed your mind when it first awakens that sets the tone for the rest of your day?

As we go through the routine of daily life, we absorb so much without even realizing it. We soak up images, tensions, energies, and experiences like a sponge. And not only the ones that belong to us—we also take in the stuff of the people around us. When we arise the next morning, we wash our bodies because we wouldn't think of starting a new day wearing yesterday's grime, but what about yesterday's psychic dirt?

Meditation washes our minds of yesterday's "stuff," clearing the slate. Just as we don't feel good if we don't wash away dirt and sweat, we also don't feel good if we don't cleanse our minds through meditation. We are not free to grow, to gain new insights and perspectives if we are weighed down by a lifetime of overreactions and emotional experiences.

There is a story of a professor who once visited a Zen master hoping to learn the secrets of Zen meditation. The master welcomed him into his home and put on a pot of tea. The professor sat and talked on and on about all he knew and all he hoped to learn. When the tea was ready, the Zen master began to pour some into the professor's cup. He poured and poured until the tea filled the cup and spilled over the brim. He kept pouring until the tea ran out onto the table and down to the floor.

"Stop!" said the professor. "The cup is full!"

"I know," said the Zen master. "That cup is you. You are so full of all you know that there is no space for anything new. I can teach you nothing."

You know how good it feels to clean out your attic, closet, or garage? Well, imagine how good it will feel to clean your mind!

How does this work? The body is a condition-response mechanism that is designed to take direction from two sources: the outer world (stimuli) and the inner world (intuition). Meditation trains the mind to respond to the truth of intuition rather than the environment, hence the external chatter quiets, our cups are emptied, and we can act according to our inner direction rather than react to what is going on around us.

For every function, whether physical or spiritual, there must be a supporting mechanism. For the intuitive function, it's the third eye center. The third eye center is located near the middle of the forehead, and is widely believed to be the body's spiritual command center. When you meditate, you bring your attention to this spot. This heightened awareness attracts energy that subsequently sparks the master glands in the brain, most notably the pituitary gland, which links your biochemical and nervous systems. New brain waves are created that stimulate the impulse of intuition. This energy ultimately awakens the innate wisdom within us.

Wisdom, however, has no use or virtue on its own. Wisdom becomes noble only when it is used to *direct our actions rightly*. This is the real secret to having a meaningful purpose in life. When we act unwisely, we live ineffectively and invite physical and spiritual suffering. But living according to our wisdom, allowing our intuition to guide our actions, is the essence of truthful living. Through meditation we learn to open up to this wisdom and live our lives in more purposeful and fulfilling ways.

Meditation for Genuine Healing

One of the most profound gifts meditation practice can give you is genuine healing—the kind of healing that goes directly to the cause rather than just soothing the effect. The method of meditation I practice and teach is not a Band-Aid or another way just to feel better temporarily—that's the equivalent of spiritual aspirin. What this method can ultimately do, if the intention is right, is allow you to see the grooves of cause and effect carved within your psyche. It affords you the opportunity not just to feel better but really to heal at your deepest levels.

In meditation, we see how the ego has been involved with everything that went wrong in our lives. We see that our intuition is the alternative, and that when we let our intuition be our guide, good begins to take shape within and around us. Problems fall away by themselves. Synchronicity takes over and things just seem to fall into place without any scheming or planning on our part. It is almost humiliating to our ego, which is used to huffing and puffing and straining to gain a result.

Living most of my life around the healing arts world has given me the opportunity to see and learn a lot about how people can and do make real and lasting changes. On the other hand, I've also seen how good many of us have gotten at staying within our comfort zones and never really changing at all, only masking the problems.

Our society has created many ways for us not to have to change our disease-centered habits. All we do is take away the pain that a certain habit or emotional circumstance is creating rather than going deeper and actually changing the root of the habit or circumstance. Let's say you suffer from headaches. You take a pill and the headache eases; hence you believe you are better. But you haven't cured the cause of your headache. You've only masked the pain. Remember what I said earlier: To truly heal, you need to feel. Within the pain are messages, information, and truths that can lead us straight into the heart of the problem.

We take care of one symptom, but then another crops up as a result of our "cure," and the next thing we know, we've got a whole new problem. We end up in more pain and therefore in need of more solutions to numb ourselves. There's a cascading effect. People tend to simply replace one problem with another. Unless this process of error is corrected, dis-ease will manifest itself in a variety of ways. Since most people don't seek health until they are sick or in pain, they are just patching up symptoms. What they really need is a wrecking ball to break out the old foundation that is full of cracks and holes and build a whole new base.

My student Ariel shared this revelation with me: Whenever her relationship wasn't going well, she would feel depressed. So she would eat chocolate to make herself feel better, but eating a lot of chocolate would cause her to gain weight and her face to break out. So then she felt worse because she wouldn't be able to fit into her clothes and would be embarrassed by her acne. She'd start working out at the gym compulsively, spending nearly an hour a day on the Stairmaster, which would strain her knees. Then she'd need to take painkillers, which would give her stomach distress. She'd take medication for her acne that would produce a whole set of negative results on its own. The cascade effect would go into full force. Each solution Ariel turned to invited its own set of new problems, which then required

new solutions, and the downward spiral into a loss of vitality became inevitable.

Though it may have been obvious to those around her, for a long time Ariel couldn't see the cycle because she was in the center of it. The original cause of the cycle was no longer the focus because she was so busy trying to fix the symptoms. For many years it never occured to her to search for growth and healing in the area of her relationship because she was fixated on her physical image problems.

Through the use of drugs (including food, which can function as a drug) we have the power to cause powerful chemical changes in the body. However, this proves not only to be temporary but also very harmful. Disease, illness, aches, pains, and distress are warnings that one of the laws of the body, mind, and soul is being violated. A quick-fix cure only masks something that needs to be made fully visible for healing.

All good things, including a yoga practice, can help you cope with life and the problems, challenges, and realities that face us. However, as I said earlier, stress management isn't our focus, transformation is. Eating healthy food, getting a massage, going for a long walk, or practicing a series of yoga poses can trigger a glandular response and therefore a chemical shift in your body. But a biological effect is not necessarily a genuine healing factor. If you feel bad and you do something that makes you feel good, you will naturally feel better and think that your condition has improved. But the point to genuine healing is that feeling better and being better are not the same.

Let's look at a yoga pose as an example—say, doing a Shoulder Stand when you feel lethargic. Shoulder Stand is an inverted position in which the body is turned upside down and the weight is supported by the shoulders and the base of the neck. The neck is tucked sharply forward in this position, shutting off a vertebral artery in the throat. This forcefully diverts the flow of blood through the thyroid, which then reactivates and massages it and its sister gland, the parathyroid. Now you feel more alive and energized. You are revitalized.

The question is, are you actually better because of this process? The answer is potentially yes and potentially no.

Yes, because the daily yoga practice and individual postures cause repatterning and rewiring of your whole physiological system. This process keeps your muscles flexible and strong, your tissue clean, your blood flowing, and your organs and glands vital.

But also no, because if a fundamental root problem has not been solved, then even your yoga practice is being used to mask symptoms. Why is the thyroid depleted in the first place? If it needed stimulation, the condition was probably a result of a lifestyle that is draining it, which resulted in an overall state of exhaustion.

When life has pinned me up against a wall or brought me to my knees, I've learned to ask, am I correcting that which really needs correcting? Remember, we are talking about meditation for truthful living! We are talking about the difference between coping with life and completely transforming our relationship to it, about asking the deeper questions rather than just superficially soothing ourselves.

Do you know why you eat the way you do, and the effects it has?
Do you give your body the true rest it needs?
Do you know why you react the way you do?
Why do you work as hard as you do?
Are you holding on to fears, resentments, anxieties?
Are you aware of why you play out the roles you do in your relationships?

It's not easy to ask or examine what lies beneath our symptoms. But as Plato said, "The life which is unexamined is not worth living." The real transformation, the real healing, the real strength, the real peace and power come from dealing with the root—the cause of anything in our life that isn't working. Learning how to differentiate such delicate points of cause and effect in your approach to life is the first step toward freeing body and soul. Meditation practice awakens the special insight, spiritual vision, and common sense that allows you to see into these nuances and subtleties. Each layer of illusion you peel away reveals new discoveries, new insights, and new opportunities for genuine healing.

Putting on Your Spiritual Armor

I try to meditate every morning and evening. When I don't, I feel it. My days just feel different. I feel less effective, less connected, more easily frustrated by little things, unable to see options. Something is just missing. But when I start my day by sitting quietly for at least ten or fifteen minutes, I've centered myself. It's like putting on spiritual armor that gives me protection from the stresses of life.

As I sit still, I'm reversing the flow of energy so that it comes from the inside out, rather than from the outside in. I know that when I start reaching for everything out there in the world—all the distractions and temptations—I am allowing the energy to flow from the outside in. I start to soak it up like a sponge. Experiences go through me, taking root and potentially growing into knots of anxiety and dis-ease. But when I meditate there is a shift. The energy starts to flow from within me out into the world, like a river streaming down from the top of a mountain.

It can be very easy to feel connected and grounded within yourself when you are home meditating; the real challenge is to carry that sense of peace and light with you as you go through your day. Without this calm center you are like a ship without a rudder, influenced by every situation, every person, every mood. This is why it is so important to meditate every day, even if it is only for a few minutes. Even ten minutes every morning shifts your consciousness for the rest of the day. And those ten minutes will very often turn to fifteen, twenty, thirty, or more. It's like physical exercise: The more you do, the more your body yearns for it. Once you taste it, you start to crave it. It begins to work, and eventually you don't want to go out into the world without it.

The Technique

As mentioned, the meditation technique I use is very simple, but within that simplicity lies its power. My experience tells me that this method works. However, as with anything, I always say that it is best to apply what makes sense to you and let the results speak for themselves, as they have for me and for thousands of my students.

The basic focus of this technique is to stay present by being aware of the fleeting thoughts in your mind, the ebb and flow of your breath, and the environment surrounding you. By stepping back inside yourself and observing your thoughts, you bring your mind from distraction to direction, from chaos to focus.

If you think it would be useful, you can take a tape recorder and read the following instructions out loud to play back when you do your practice. You can make whatever revisions or additions you would like to personalize the process and make it meaningful for you, though I encourage you to keep the basic structure.

Sit in whatever position is comfortable for you, as long as you can maintain a straight spine. I don't recommend lying down, because it is too easy to fall asleep, and it is important that you remain awake and alert. Place your hands in your lap in a prayerlike position, thumbs facing up, your fingertips touching and your palms gently coming apart. Close your eyes and just come into your body.

Set your intention that there is no greater place to be than right here, right now. Let go of any head stuff that keeps you from being in the present. Let go of expectations. Drop your mask and be receptive to whatever comes up. Stop trying and doing and just come into a true and deep sense of surrender.

Bring attention to your base. Feel the floor, chair, pillow, or whatever it is you are sitting on. Just notice your base. And then gently walk the fingers of your mind up your spine to the top of your head.

Now, with your eyes still closed, look through the center of your forehead. Don't look with the pupils of your eyes, use instead your mind's eye. It is as though you were stepping back into the middle of your mind and looking at the inside of your own head. You may see flashes of light, you may see colors, or you may see total darkness. Whatever you see, simply notice it. Just watch the inner wall of your forehead as if you were sitting in the middle of a room

and watching one of the four walls. Now bring your attention to your hands and rest your attention on them. Soon they will feel warm and start to tingle. Whenever we bring awareness to any point of our anatomy we are moving energy in that direction, so it will physically become warm. Don't force your attention on your hands, just feel and watch them with your mind's eye. Feel the energy flowing into your hands. Bring awareness to your thumbs, your first fingers, second fingers, third fingers, and fourth fingers. Shift your attention from one finger to another until your connection is steady. Make them glow with the calm power of your focused mind.

Funneling your awareness to your hands bridges your mind and body and brings you to the present moment. We are using your body as an anchor for your mind. Whenever you feel your mind start to wander (and it will wander!), just return your attention to your hands and begin again. Meditation is an unending process of beginning again. If your mind pulls you into forgetfulness and you slip into past or future thoughts, simply remember this moment and begin again by bring your attention back to your hands. Now radiate your awareness into and throughout your whole body. Be perfectly present and perfectly relaxed. Sense your body's presence in the room as though someone else was watching you. Notice the contact of your clothing on your skin. Observe the outline of your body, its blueprint.

Bring your awareness to your breath: to

the ebb and flow, in and out of your nostrils. Watch it rise and fall, mentally noting the in and out of every inhalation and exhalation. Don't try to change or control the breath, just observe it as it is.

Open your ears and hear every sound in the room. Simply let every noise flow in one ear and out the other. Hearing grounds you in moment-to-moment awareness. It brings you into the here and now, and the being present to each "now" moment is the essence of mindfulness. When you hear the sounds around you, simply listen without manufacturing or creating any thoughts around them.

Begin to notice your thoughts. By this simple act you step outside your thoughts into the role of observer and increase the space between them. The light shines through the space, widening the gap between stimulus and response and giving more time and space for intuitive responses to arise. In our normal state of consciousness, we come to believe we are our thoughts. But **you are not your thoughts!** If you can observe them, then clearly they are something separate from you. Each time you become aware that you are thinking, you have slammed on the brakes and entered new mental territory, a new field of consciousness.

Notice every thought that tries to steal your attention. Just notice it and bring your attention back to your hands, your body's blueprint, your breath, your senses. Don't follow your thoughts into the stream of dream stuff. What tends to happen is that we have a thought, and before we know it, we start building a story around it. Thoughts come up and they carry us away. Maybe you flash to what you had for dinner. You think about the angel food cake you had for dessert. Then your mind goes to devil's food cake, which reminds you of grandma. And then you remember it's grandma's birthday next week and you have to get a card, which makes you realize you have to stop at the bank . . . and on and on it goes. You've built an entire story around one little thought.

Don't struggle to free yourself from your thoughts. Just become aware of them. As soon as you become conscious that you have become involved with mental chatter, you've freed yourself from it. Just bring your attention gently back to your hands and let the thought go as quickly as it came in. Beginning again and again is the whole act of meditation practice. Over and over, we begin again. Let it all be natural, no manipulation. Just be here and now, breathing and observing your thoughts and letting go.

When you first start to sit, your mind will be all over the map. Thoughts will race to the surface—it may feel like chaos in your head. A torrent of thoughts, plans, conversations, anxieties, aches and pains, even musical rhythms will come flooding up. Your mind is like a whitewater river. There is a constant stream of sinkholes that are trying to suck you in and currents that fight to whisk you away from the present moment. If you happen to get caught in the rapids of your thought stream, don't fight it. Simply step out of the current onto the shore and watch as the river of thoughts flows by you. Relax and come back into your body and breath.

You may feel fidgety, uncomfortable, ready to scream or jump up and leave the room. Your ego may say, "Thanks, but no thanks. This may be great for some people, but definitely not for me." Recognize that this is all resistance! Just let go and begin again. Emotions may bubble up to the surface for review and release. Don't struggle to contain them or react. Stay in your body and even have a little cry if you need to. Feel your feelings without losing yourself in the sadness, fear, pain, or grief. Let go and let good flow in, and begin again.

Sit in this practice for at least ten minutes and work your way up to forty-five. Like yoga practice, it's better to do a little bit often rather than a whole lot once in a while. The time will increase naturally as you are ready. If you get caught up with counting minutes, just set a timer or alarm clock so you are released from having to worry about how long you have been sitting.

I encourage you to meditate every day, once in the morning and once at night. If you sit for even ten minutes every morning, you will feel a difference. Over time, your level of awareness will continue to rise so that you see people, places, and things in a whole new way. You will be given a new vision, so to speak. You will see the cause of suffering in your life and intuitively know what you need to do to begin to live in better, more fulfilling ways. You will begin to live from cause rather than effect, from within the harmony of your inner knowing rather than the chaos of your mind. Meditation isn't the magical way to the light, but it certainly is the way to the Way. Start your practice and watch the path unfold!

How to Cultivate a Daily Meditation Practice

Plan to meditate at about the same time every day. You can do it as soon as you get up in the morning, in the afternoon, and/or in the evening before bed.

Sit as long as you can every day. An ideal session is twenty to thirty minutes, but even five minutes twice a day will connect you.

Determine before you sit how long you will meditate. This will prevent your ego from diverting your initial intention.

Keep it simple. The purpose is not to induce a state of mind but to bring a new dimension of awareness and perspective to your daily experiences.

Let go of expectations. Be open and receptive to what comes up. Let go of judgments and the head stuff that keeps you from being present.

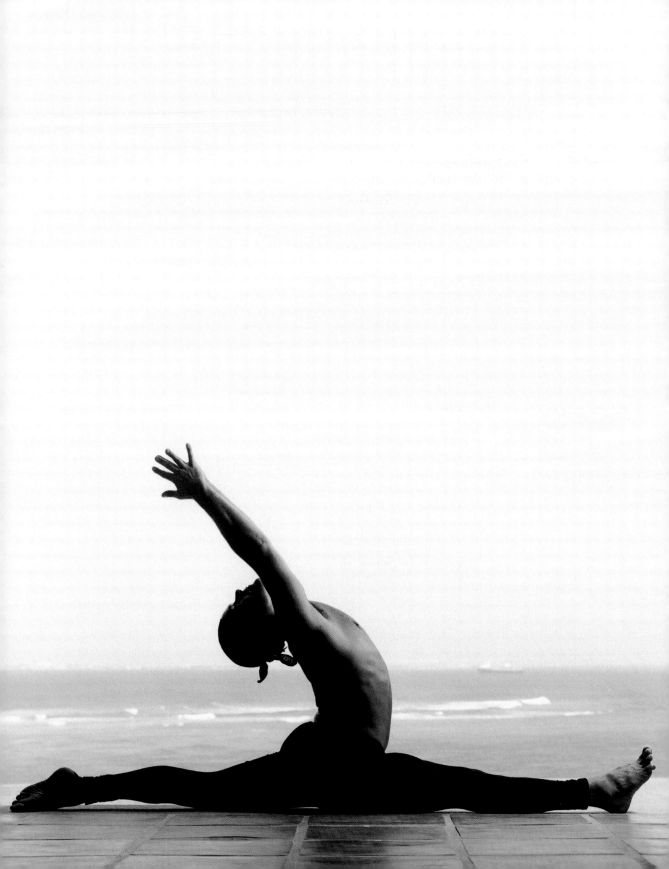

Every spirit builds itself a house, and beyond its
house a world, and beyond its world a heaven.

—Ralph Waldo Emerson

PART 5

Journeying into
Real Life

ON A RECENT TRIP TO LOS ANGELES, I
WENT TO ONE OF MY OLD HAUNTS, GOLD'S GYM, IN
VENICE BEACH. THAT PARTICULAR GYM IS LIKE THE WORLD MECCA OF

bodybuilding. Arnold trained there, as have countless others. When I told a friend where I'd gone, she laughed and said, "I love it . . . the big yogi pumps iron?"

"It's all yoga," I told her. "On or off the mat, it's yoga."

Even if I'm in the crème de la crème of the weightlifting world, I'm still putting all I have learned in my practice into action. I'm using my ujjayi breathing for stamina and presence, my abdominal lock for core stabilization, a focused gaze for calm determination, the Master Principles of Alignment for healthy form. Yes, I'm lifting weights, but beyond that I stay aware of my edge, practice maintaining equanimity,

and use my intuition to know when less is more and when to push further.

Yoga isn't just about what happens on the mat. It is so much more than postures, or meditation in motion, or breathing, or eating to cleanse. If this whole program didn't have a practical, real-life value, I wouldn't bother living or teaching it—that would be a waste of time. What all of this is really about is total life transformation. It's what happens in every waking moment: using your intuition as your guide to change any circumstance in your life.

The true Journey into Power means living the practices and principles I have been talking about in every dimension of your life: your body, your spirit, your work, your relationships, your environment. All the tools in this book are the means for you to wake up, discover your connection to the power of the universe, and transform your body, your life, and the world from the inside out.

The real essence of power is the energy that is within and behind us. You already know that there is a force **within** you that is not necessarily **of** you. This magnificent force, which runs the universe, is always there, willing to support you; let go and allow that force to guide your actions. This force whispers to you in the language of intuition, and it is your intuition that allows you to live from your authentic self.

As we rewire our minds toward true growth, we can let go of our attachment to money, popularity, prestige, and all the things we strive for in this world, because in our hearts we now know that by themselves these things will lead us nowhere. We can stop chasing what we once perceived as success and let a natural unfolding occur.

As we meditate and learn to move, breathe, and be from our calm center, we become new men and women. We become open vessels through which the universe can channel light, truth, and love. Continually refining our practice and our purposeful intention allows us to radiate a power in this world that is not of this world. People will not fail to notice, and we will be repaid in many ways and on may levels unseen.

If we do our part, the universe will infuse us with all things good. It really comes down to that simple principle. The more you honor and respect your body, your self, your life, and those around you, the greater the rewards you will receive in return. The more we shine the light of consciousness into every dark corner of our minds, the greater our ability to see things in new ways. The more we release old attitudes, face the fire, forgive, and open our hearts, the greater insights we receive. And the more we integrate all aspects of our existence into one flow of intention toward growth, the more our lives begin to flow. As you mature spiritually, you come to truly appreciate, trust, and surrender to the light that is within you, and from there, you can do anything!

Maintaining the Meditative Mind State

Imagine this: You wake up in the morning, meditate, and do your yoga practice before starting your day. You feel peaceful as you go about your morning, taking a shower, reading the paper, eating breakfast. You head outside or wherever your car is parked and discover that someone has put a huge dent in the driver's-side door. You react automatically and immediately, getting annoyed and angry, and suddenly—*bam!*—your peace goes to pieces. The equanimity you found just a few minutes before vanishes when you are confronted with the stress of everyday life.

The practices in this book will do you no good whatsoever if you roll up and put away the meditative mind state along with your yoga mat. What good is being calm and centered for one hour a day if you are going to abandon your spirit for the other twenty-three? The Bhagavad Gita—the "yogic bible"—is one big metaphysical war story in which the student warrior trains his mind and heart with yogic disciplines; cultivates virtue, wisdom, and clarity; and then goes out and fights on the battlefield. Your practice helps you to rise above the mental battlefields—both of this world and of your mind. If you've ever been to one of my classes, you've heard me say, "Your real practice begins when you leave class." Living from equanimity and your calm center of dignity is something you need to strive for twenty-four hours a day, not just a few hours a week.

The mini-crises that occur from day to day can serve as fertilizer for your growth. They reveal lessons to learn, patterns to break, reactions to become aware of, resistance to break through. Stress isn't always pleasant, but it definitely enriches your spiritual soil! It's not necessarily only big things that upset our inner balance; the accumulation of reactions to small things is also a factor. Overreactive people are impacted and imprinted by their environment, soaking up all the stresses and pressures like a sponge and storing them in muscles and mind. They are often supersensitive to their physical environment. If the weather is good, they feel good. If it isn't, their attitude and way of being is diminished. They are also influenced by "social weather." When people treat them well, they feel good; when people don't, they become depressed, defensive, or even sick. Reactive and insecure people build their emotional lives around the behavior of others.

Part of our journey is learning how to carry our own weather with us, so no matter if it rains or shines, we don't lose our ability to be patient, kind, and come from a place of love rather than resentment. We can respond from a place of patience and respect regardless of what happens around us. We are then "in" formed—formed from within—rather than formed by outside forces.

Someone once asked Gandhi, "If you want to be with God, why don't you go live in a Himalayan cave?" Gandhi replied, "If I thought God was in a Himalayan cave I would go there immediately, but I believe God is found in humanity."

We don't need to give it all up and go live in a cave somewhere to maintain our meditative mind state. My father used to say that if you put an exotic flower in a hothouse, it thrives, but if you put it out on a street in New York City, it will wilt in minutes. Anyone can be yogic in an ashram. But can you bring that into real life?

Your practice brings you to your center of dignity, to the objective state of equanimity where light, patience, and true love are found. So how do you protect the meditative mind-set in the middle of conflict?

Live the principles you employ on your yoga mat.

Practice daily to strengthen your inner light.

See conflict without resenting it or wanting to change it.

Look at the conflict in front of you straight in the eye. Don't be a doormat! Stand firm without becoming reactive.

Know that it doesn't matter if people love you in that moment; you love them. It doesn't matter if people understand you; you understand them. And if they do not forgive you, you forgive them.

Be patient under trial. As long as you are not judgmental or resentful, you will be able to disagree without being disagreeable.

If you have something to say, say it. Don't be upset or react; just say it.

If you have something to do, do it. Don't be upset or react; just do it with presence.

Don't be overly excited by praise or offended by criticism. And don't be too quick to give praise or criticism.

Don't take things personally. Remember, it's usually not about you.

Always follow your intuition.

Practice doubting your doubts when they arise.

Do not fall into the trap of competition and comparison.

Stay in your body in moments of adversity.

Let go and have faith in the power of the universe. It is always there for you, all you ever need to do is let go and let it in!

The Ripple Effect

Platonic philosophy talks about life being like a wheel. At the center of the wheel is an energy that floods out into all the spokes of our lives. We tend to separate everything in our lives into categories— our work is over here, our relationships are over there, and somewhere else is our health and spiritual life. But really, everything is connected to everything else. This deeper level of integration is the next step on your journey, where your body, soul, and lifestyle are all interwoven as one. You know your practice is working when every interaction in your life flows forth from this oneness.

When you go deeper into your heart, your truth naturally fans out into all the areas of your life. As your transformation unfolds, you may start to look around and question your work, your relationships, what you say and do. When you awaken the charisma of authenticity within you, it is natural to start to look at your life and see it with entirely new eyes.

You may notice times and situations in which you are not speaking your truth. Where before you might have been able to gloss over these moments, perhaps now you feel uncomfortable doing so. You live your truth by sharing it, and to the extent that you are withholding it from others, you are denying yourself. Don't be afraid to speak your truth. If delivered from the heart with kindness, honesty, and genuine intent, the effects can be astonishing and can take life, health, and relationships to new levels. It may not necessarily be easy to speak from the heart—you may ruffle some feathers—but as you continue to cultivate your equanimity and meditative mind state, it will come more naturally. You will become less concerned with pleasing others and avoiding conflict and more focused on living joyously and freely from your truth, come what may.

You may become aware that some relationships are no longer serving you, or that certain situations do not reflect your core values. Lilly, a longtime student of mine, came to a Bootcamp in Montana. She was meditating on the top of a mountain and came to the sad but profound realization that she did not want to marry her fiancé, whom she knew deep in her heart was not right for her. Another student who worked on Wall Street used to go to happy hour every day after work with his colleagues and smoke and drink right through dinner. After he came to a Mexico Bootcamp, he decided he no longer wanted to take part in that kind of toxic lifestyle. His colleagues gave him a hard time, but he remained committed to his choice. Friends or loved ones may not understand when you change like this, but if you stay calmly aligned with what is true for you, that change will lead you to a real and authentic place within your life.

You may feel drawn to examine your life's work—either the path you have chosen or the energy you put behind it. A student at a workshop told the group that once she started to practice regularly, she no longer wanted to produce the negative political campaign ads that had been her job for several years. She wanted to use her talents to spread hope, not cynicism.

Your work in the world is meant to be about expressing the power and spirit that's within you. It's not necessarily about the specific job you do or the position you hold. Whether you are a missionary or a bricklayer, a schoolteacher or the CEO of a major corporation, what matters is that you show up with complete presence and magnificence. It is the power of your personal contribution that creates true prosperity, wealth, and abundance for you and all those around you.

Continuing Your Practice

The Journey into Power is a lifelong practice. As you grow and evolve in your own way, your practice will grow and evolve. It will be different from day to day, week to week, year to year. What matters the most is that you just continue to show up and do it.

You can seek out little tips and tricks for staying motivated, but what it comes down to is intention. It's not *how* you do something that empowers you. It's *why* you are doing it. What do you want for yourself? Is there another reality that would be more fulfilling, more authentic, more truthful? Do you want to just cope with the stresses of life, or do you want to rise above them? Do you want to survive, or do you want to radiate? How far do you want to go?

We all know the saying "If you know better, do better." It's simple: If we live and do what we know is right in our hearts, we grow. Living what you know creates a state of being that I call "clicking," in which everything in your life just effortlessly clicks into place and you live in forward momentum. Daily practice keeps you plugged in and keeps that forward momentum happening. Maintain your practice by doing a little bit a lot and that will be your anchor in life.

Once you are inwardly changed and your growth is the central focus of your life, falling off track is not an option. It might happen, but your conscience will scream louder than ever. In those moments, the light shows you the way back and you simply begin anew.

Shining On

You don't need permission to shine. That's the biggest mistake we make in life; we think we need someone's approval to be magnificent or to just own what is true to us. But we are all not only capable of radiating light and love, it is our moral responsibility.

A part of our maturing and venturing into authentic power is putting aside all small and worthless values. The world needs this from us at this time. It used to be an option to grow and to be present. But personal strength and presence of mind is no longer a luxury, it is an absolute necessity. Our families need us to be present, our communities need us to be present, the world needs us to be present.

Being true to your inner knowing is one of the most precious gifts you can give to the people around you. I remember when I first started teaching yoga from my heart, people loved my classes. I didn't really know the "right" way to teach, but I had a lot of fun. People used to come up to me after a class and say, "That was so amazing . . . I'll be back!" My class size grew like crazy. I didn't know all the rules of teaching, but I knew how to show up fully and give what I had. It felt good, natural, and right. This went on for a couple of years, and then a terrible thing happened.

A famous yoga teacher who I really admired sat down with me and said, "You know, Baron, you are a good teacher, but you don't have any formal training. Let me train you."

A sense of self-doubt overtook me, and I started scrambling to learn all the rules. I thought if I could get the rules down, then maybe I wouldn't just be a good teacher, I'd be a great one. So I listened and learned from good teachers all the principles of how to teach and do it right. I tried to sound the way I thought a yoga teacher should sound, and doing what a "good" yoga teacher does. People stopped coming to my classes because suddenly the spirit, the energy, and the charisma of what I had been doing was lost. Suddenly I wasn't fun anymore. When the joy was lost for me, the depletion of my personal power set in, and the magic in my classroom was lost.

It didn't take long before I stopped trying to be who I was "supposed" to be. I threw away my doubts about who I truly was and went back to teaching from my heart. Attendance surged again, and I learned a very valuable lesson. I realized that I had educated myself right out of my common sense and innocence—what some call beginner's luck. It's a mistake that I will never repeat. I now know that if you truly believe in the presence within you, the love in your heart will guide you and you'll naturally flow from your inner light. Just show up, shine, and be yourself at whatever you are called to do. If you do that, you will be great!

If you listen to successful people who made their dreams come true, you see that they followed their hearts and made their own rules. We can follow the rules, and they may help us—we may even grow to a degree—but eventually we need to break out of the box and rediscover our innocence. What makes your heart sing? Within that question is the key to expressing, sharing, and making your ultimate contribution to this earth.

At the end of every Bootcamp, as I look around at the glowing faces, I tell my students, "Go forth and shine; go bless the world." It is not enough just to awaken within yourself and your own life. As my father taught me so many years ago when he encouraged me to teach my very first class, you need to share your light with those around you. The wealthiest place on the planet is not a gold or diamond mine, or even a palace. It is our graveyards, because so many people die with their brilliance, gifts, and talents inside. They did not share who they were with anyone, perhaps not even with themselves.

The next step after self-fulfillment is making a contribution to the world. This can take on many different forms and will be deeply personal to you. Maybe you choose to make small changes in the way you relate to the people around you, even strangers. Maybe you choose to be more generous with your money, time, or energy. Maybe you step up and contribute to your community, or maybe you can just be an example to the people around you. As Gandhi said, "You must be the change you wish to see in the world."

Have you been living your truth in your body, your mind, your soul, and the world? If you haven't, then the good news is that the mystery is solved as to why you don't have what you want on this earth. Armed with the knowledge you've gleaned from this book, you *can* have what you really want!

It is so, so simple: We get what we give. If we respect our bodies, they will be our vessels for transformation. If we put forth honesty, sincerity, and love, we will receive them in return. And if we don't like what we've been doing, then the beautiful thing to remember is that we can always start over again. Just as the meditation practice teaches, we simply begin again. This is a journey with no end, with many paths and many turns along the way.

If you find yourself walking down the wrong path, simply change direction and begin again.

We are surrounded with opportunities to grow and fuel our Journey into Power. We are powerful when we open our spiritual eyes and ears and really dare to be fully present. We are powerful when we live and share from our hearts rather than from the chaos in our heads. We are powerful when we exceed ourselves and find our exceeding selves. We radiate power when we speak our truth, come what may. When we live at cause and from truth, the heights and depths to which we may journey are infinite.

The great teacher Rama Krishna once said, "The winds of grace are blowing all the time. All we need to do is raise our sails." I hope you raise your sails high and journey forward into your best life.

Namaste.

Resources

Congratulations! You've taken the first step. Now—continue the extraordinary journey into the soul of strength and serenity, and expand your personal and spiritual power! Let Baron Baptiste's tools of transformation show you how.

Baptiste Power Yoga Institute's mission is to bring yoga to as many people as possible as a path of transformation to a healthier, happier, and more powerful life. We are not just offering "yoga as usual"; we develop and design our products, programs, and classes so that they are relevant to your every waking moment and accessible for all levels of abilities, ages, and interests. If you have an interest in taking this powerful process to the next level, you can start with the basic step of purchasing a product, or if you want to take a deep plunge into radical, invigorating change you can come to one of our weekend or weeklong programs.

Videos, DVDs, Audio CDs, and Yoga Products

We've created our video and audio products as a way for you to take the transformational process home or on the road. Baptiste Power Yoga is based on intuition rather than tradition. If you think you need to go to a health club to be wonderfully fit and beautiful, think again. If you think that you need to escape to a cave in the Himalayas to find the enlightenment that yoga promises, think again. Baptiste Yoga stretches the meaning of yoga beyond its familiar poses and breathing techniques to include a philosophy of facing life with a renewed personal force that is fueled by a deep sense of inner stillness. Our products are the ideal way for you to take Baptiste Power Yoga with you wherever you go. Visit www.baronbaptiste.com or call 1-800-936-9642 for the latest products.

Journey into Power
    Personal Training System—LIVE!
Experience the power of Baron
    on Video, DVD, and Audio CD!

Journey into Power Live! is a line of video, DVD, and audio products based on the yoga Bootcamp experience explained in this book; these programs take the principles of this book and help you put them into action. In these powerful programs, Baron will take you through a transformation of your body and mind. All products include a variety of modifications so that you may practice exactly where you are regardless of experience. Anyone can do them, from the absolute beginner to the seasoned practitioner. You'll be taken step by step through a power vinyasa yoga flow; you'll be guided through a powerful meditation session to create important changes in your life and to establish greater serenity and inner strength in your every waking moment; you'll learn the simple keys to vibrant health and energy and the principles of eating to fuel your body and not your ego. All it takes is a simple intention—that you want your life to change, to grow, to evolve. Call us at 1-800-936-9642 or visit www.baronbaptiste.com for more information.

Journey into Power Live! Workshops were the source of inspiration for this book. We conduct these life-changing workshops over a series of weekends or during a seven-day Bootcamp. Attending one of these programs is an opportunity to invigorate your life through a highly dynamic combination of power vinyasa yoga, meditation for truthful living, the cleansing diet principles for a vital life, rewiring your mind, and having tons of fun in beautiful and potent locations. We have witnessed it work on thousands of people—from all over the world, with all levels of abilities, and of all ages. It is one way to charge your life, free your body, and ignite your spirit like never before.

This is much more than just a vacation. The focus is on true transformation. In our programs we create a sanctuary for your body and soul where you engage in a yogic process to enliven at every level. This is your revelation waiting to happen!

Call us at 1-800-936-9642 or visit www.baronbaptiste.com for more information on what programs we are currently offering.

The Baron Baptiste Live!
Video and DVD Series
With the soul-stirring music
    of Krishna Das

Soul of Strength—Light, Free, and Energized
The Soul of Strength is an easy-to-follow 60-minute yoga practice designed for any age, weight, or fitness level! You'll receive detailed explanations of each move and extensive tips on proper form while the on-screen students provide demos at different

levels of intensity and ability. The brisk pace provides an excellent cardiovascular workout. Baron will inspire, encourage, and challenge you and the Live! class through the yoga process of energizing, strengthening, and healing your body and mind.

Core Power—Abs, Back, and Bliss

Core Power is an easy-to-follow 30-minute yoga practice designed for any age, weight, or fitness level! You'll alternate abdominal sculpting with simple back strengthening and lengthening postures to create a more toned, balanced, and strong center. Zero in on your abdominals, strengthen your back, and learn to move from this "power center" of your body.

Unlocking Athletic Power—Sweat, Serenity, and Sport

Unlocking Athletic Power is an easy-to-follow 30-minute yoga practice designed as the ultimate conditioning program for fitness and sports enthusiasts! You'll follow a proven method Baron has used with hundreds of professional athletes in such sports as football, basketball, golf, racquetball, and tennis. Baron guides you through a practice that targets the "core" muscle groups of the abdominals and the back, and gives special focus to the essential muscles of the hips and pelvis. You'll develop a flexible strength and move with a new sense of physical freedom, agility, and grace.

Baron Baptiste Live! Power Vinyasa Yoga and Meditation Audio CDs

- *Putting Postures to Your Prayers* (Audio CD)
- *Bodyprayers* (Audio CD)
- *The Soul of Flow* (Audio CD)
- *The Soul of Strength & Serenity* (Audio CD)
- *Journey into Power: The Practice* (Audio CD)
- *Meditation for Beginners* (Audio CD)
- *Journey into the Power of Meditation* (Audio CD)

Putting Postures to Your Prayers, Body Prayers, The Soul of Flow, The Soul of Strength & Serenity, and Journey into Power are easy-to-use 75-minute Power Yoga practices on audio CD designed for any age, weight, or fitness level! Baron will inspire, encourage, and challenge you and the live classroom of students through the yoga process of energizing, strengthening, and healing your body and mind. It's as if you are right in the middle of a class with Baron. You'll receive detailed explanations of each move and extensive tips on proper form. In a seamless manner, the practice is broken down into separate tracks. So you can choose to do the complete flow, or if pressed for time, choose the tracks and design your workout. Get ready to feel the power!

Journey into the Power of Meditation and Meditation for Beginners with Baron Baptiste give you a "road map" to help you along the path to greater intuition, equanimity, and freedom from stress. In these 30-minute CDs, Baron will guide you through a simple meditation exercise that will release emotional, psychological, and physical blocks. You'll learn how to use this powerful technique to enter "the zone" whenever you want. This practical tool will pave the way for inner and outer transformation. These programs show you how to remove everyday irritations and worries from your life, replace stress with deep inner calm, and gain a new sense of inner strength and personal power.

Call us at 1-800-936-9642 or visit www.baronbaptiste.com.

Baptiste Power Yoga Studios

The Baptiste Power Vinyasa Yoga Studios are built on a simple principle: that everyone can do yoga, regardless of age, strength, or weight. Our classes will lead you to building and maintaining a physical and spiritual vitality, which will change your life completely.

Each Baptiste studio offers our classic All-levels and Power Yoga Basic classes for students of different levels of experience and fitness abilities. We teach a practice with a solid physical base coupled with an intellectual understanding in which to continue your journey into power! Attending our classes will expand your spiritual understanding while helping you to build strength, stamina, flexibility, focus, and a renewed personal force. Attending classes at our studios three times a week will establish the flow in your life. Attending class five to six times a week will transform your existence.

Visit www.baronbaptiste.com or call 1-800-936-9642 for studio locations.

Teacher Training Programs

If you are ready to take a bold step in your life and enter the flow at a totally different angle, consider one of our Teacher Training Programs. We offer weekend and weeklong intensive Teacher Training Bootcamps for those aspiring to teach the Journey into Power Principles and Baptiste Power Yoga.

Baron Baptiste's teachers' programs are an exclusive hands-on opportunity for you, if you wish to hone your ability to transform the lives of individuals seeking physical and spiritual growth, leading them to a healthier state of existence. We establish an amazing learning environment in which you can challenge yourself like never before. You won't just learn skills "intellectually"—you'll put them into practice immediately, achieving incredible results that will stay with you forever. You'll learn more, do more, achieve more, transform more than anyone could reasonably expect, and grow more than you could ever imagine. Call us at 1-800-936-9642 or visit www.baronbaptiste.com for more information on our current Teacher Trainings schedule.

The Baptiste Foundation

The Baptiste Foundation is a not-for-profit organization focused on bringing the transformational power of yoga and meditation to individuals and communities in need. Whether someone is fighting an addiction, rebuilding a life, struggling financially, or living a challenged physical life, the Baptiste Foundation is built on the belief that *when one applies the timeless principles of authentic living to their life* then one can transcend one's struggles, bringing light to darkness and success to all aspects of one's life.

In our present world, filled with violence, personal turbulence, and anger, there is an urgent call ringing out for contribution fueled by love and timeless understanding that has the strength to make this world a better place. It is the Baptiste Foundation's mission to discover new, innovative paths to continue our journey of shedding light on each and every person we reach. As our light grows, so does the light of the world.

Visit www.baronbaptiste.com for more information.

However you choose, whether through a product or a journey, we hope that your journey is one of constant growth and truth. Remember, it is a process—and you have the ability to do it right now!

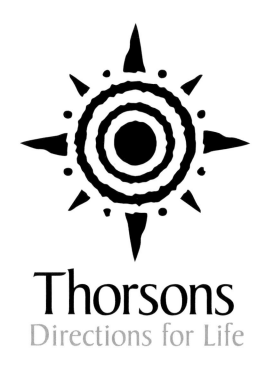

Thorsons
Directions for Life

This online sanctuary is packed with information, inspiration and guidance to help you on the path to physical and spiritual well-being. Drawing on the integrity and vision of our authors and titles, and with health advice, articles, astrology, tarot, a meditation zone, author interviews and events listings, Thorsons.com is a great alternative to help create space and peace in our lives.

So if you've always wondered about practising yoga, following an allergy-free diet, using the tarot or getting a life coach, we can point you in the right direction.

Make www.thorsons.com your online sanctuary.

www.thorsons.com